Winningham and *Preusser's*
CRITICAL THINKING CASES in NURSING
Fourth Edition

medical-surgical, pediatric, maternity, and psychiatric case studies

Barbara A. Preusser, PhD, FNPc

Family Nurse Practitioner
Veterans Administration Medical Center
Salt Lake City, Utah

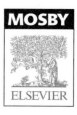
MOSBY
ELSEVIER

11830 Westline Industrial Drive
St. Louis, Missouri 63146

WINNINGHAM AND PREUSSER'S CRITICAL THINKING CASES IN NURSING: MEDICAL-SURGICAL, PEDIATRIC, MATERNITY, AND PSYCHIATRIC CASE STUDIES, FOURTH EDITION   ISBN: 978-0-323-05359-4

Notice

Knowledge and best practice in this field are constantly changing. As new research and experience broaden our knowledge, changes in practice, treatment and drug therapy may become necessary or appropriate. Readers are advised to check the most current information provided (i) on procedures featured or (ii) by the manufacturer of each product to be administered, to verify the recommended dose or formula, the method and duration of administration, and contraindications. It is the responsibility of the practitioner, relying on his or her own experience and knowledge of the patient, to make diagnoses, to determine dosages and the best treatment for each individual patient, and to take all appropriate safety precautions. To the fullest extent of the law, neither the Publisher nor the Author assumes any liability for any injury and/or damage to persons or property arising out of or related to any use of the material contained in this book.

The Publisher

Library of Congress Control Number: 2008922011

ISBN: 978-0-323-05359-4

Acquisitions Editor: Kristin Geen
Senior Developmental Editor: Lauren K. Lake
Publishing Services Manager: Deborah L. Vogel
Senior Project Manager: Deon Lee
Senior Book Designer: Amy Buxton

Printed in the United States of America

Last digit is the print number: 9 8 7 6 5 4 3 2

To Maryl L. Winningham, APRN, PhD, FACSM,
who died February 18, 2001, from complications of breast cancer.

Dr. Winningham shared with her surviving Co-Editor, Dr. Barbara Preusser, a singular commitment to the ideal of excellence in nursing practice.

The educational philosophy that informs and underlies this text and that drove the effort to publish it was held in common between Maryl and Barbara. Their core educational philosophy can be summed up in the following statement: "Errors in a safe environment."

To this day, it remains the view of the author that a case studies approach to nursing education creates a situation in which students can make and learn from their mistakes without jeopardizing patients. It is our hope that students who use this text will strive as diligently for truly professional compassion as they do for technical excellence in the care they administer to their patients.

Frederick Kesler

Clinical Consultants

Pharmacy
Rae Murphy, RPh
Salt Lake City, Utah

Nutrition
Linda J. Winningham, MS, RD
Saline, Michigan

Reviewer
Frederick Kesler
Salt Lake City, Utah

Contributors

Elizabeth Jane Bell, MSN, ANPc
Pulmonary Clinic
Veterans Administration Medical Center
Salt Lake City, Utah

Lesley A. Black, BSN, MS, ANPc, CWOCN
Urology Clinic
Veterans Administration Medical Center
Salt Lake City, Utah

Kent Blad, MS, FNPc, ACNP-C, FCCM
Associate Professor
Brigham Young University
Provo, Utah

Jamie Clinton-Lont, BSN, FNPc
Women's Clinic/Primary Care Clinic
Veterans Administration Medical Center
Salt Lake City, Utah

Susan L. Croft, BSN, MS
Retired Assistant Professor, Maternal-Infant
   Department
University of Utah, College of Nursing
Salt Lake City, Utah

Joyce Foster, PhD, CNM, FACNM, FAAN
Professor Emeritus, Graduate Nurse
   Midwifery Program
University of Utah, College of Nursing
Salt Lake City, Utah

Shellagh Gutke, BSN, CWOCN
Wound and Ostomy Care
Veterans Administration Medical Center
Salt Lake City, Utah

Nancy Hayden, MSN, FNPc
Urology Associates
Nashville, Tennessee

Sondra Heaston, MS, FNPc, CEN
Assistant Professor
Brigham Young University
Provo, Utah

Janice Hulbert, RN, MS
Community Health Program
Veterans Administration Medical Center

Lisa Jensen, BSN, MS, APRN, CS
Psychiatric Mental Health
Veterans Administration Medical Center
Salt Lake City, Utah

**Stephanie C. Kettendorf, MS, RN, CNS,
   NCBF**
Assistant Professor
Mount Carmel College of Nursing
Columbus, Ohio

Contributors

Julie Killebrew, BSN, MS
Associate Professor
Weber State College
Oncology Nurse
Intermountain Health Care
Ogden, Utah

Karen Kone, BSN, ACRN
HIV Nurse Educator, Liver Transplant
  Coordinator
Veterans Administration Medical Center
Salt Lake City, Utah

Kathleen Kuntz, MSN, APRN, SANE
Women Veteran Program Manager
Veterans Administration Medical Center
Salt Lake City, Utah

Janet G. Madsen, PhD
Clinical Psychologist
Veterans Administration Medical Center
Salt Lake City, Utah

Debra Ann Mills, RN, MS
Associate Teaching Professor
Brigham Young University, College of
  Nursing
Provo, Utah

Jeanie O'Donnell, MSN
Renal Clinic
Veterans Administration Medical Center
Salt Lake City, Utah

Deb Plasman-Coles, PAc
Gastrointestinal Clinic
Granger Medical Center
West Valley City, Utah

Laura Lee Scott, MSN, FNPc
Primary Care Clinic
Veterans Administration Medical Center
Salt Lake City, Utah

Mary Seegmiller, MSN
Case Management Admissions Assessment
  Coordinator
Intermountain Health Care
Salt Lake City, Utah

Sandra Smeeding, MS, FNPc
Associate Director of Integrative Health Care
Veterans Administration Medical Center
Salt Lake City, Utah

Deborah D. Smith, BSN
Anticoagulation Clinic
Veterans Administration Medical Center
Salt Lake City, Utah

Ann Speirs, BSN
Cardiovascular Step-down
Intermountain Health Care
Salt Lake City, Utah

Ronald Ulberg, BSN, MSN
Assistant Professor
Brigham Young University
Provo, Utah

Kristy Vankatwyk, MSN, FNPc
Cardiology Clinic
Veterans Administration Medical Center
Salt Lake City, Utah

Annette S. Wendel, BSN
Educator, Oncology and Bone Marrow
  Transplant Unit
Intermountain Health Care
Salt Lake City, Utah

Wendy Whitney, MSN, FNPc, CANP
Surgical Intensive Care Unit
Veterans Administration Medical Center
Salt Lake City, Utah

Mary Youtsey, BSN, CDE
Diabetes Educator, Primary Care Clinic
Veterans Administration Medical Center
Salt Lake City, Utah

Introduction

There is an urgent need for nurses with well-practiced critical thinking skills. As new graduates you will be expected to make decisions and take actions of an increasingly sophisticated nature. You will encounter problems you have never seen or heard about during your classroom and clinical experiences. You are going to have to make complex decisions with little or no guidance and limited resources.

We want you to be exposed to as much as possible during your student days, but more importantly, we want you to learn to *think*. You cannot memorize your way out of any situation, but you can *think* your way out of any situation. We know that students often learn more and faster when they have the freedom to make mistakes. This book is designed to allow you to experiment with finding answers without the pressure of someone's life hanging in the balance. We want you to do well. We want you to be the best. It is our wish for you to grow into confident, competent professionals. After all, someday we will be one of those people you care for, and when that day comes, we want you to be very, very good at what you do!

What Is Critical Thinking?

Critical thinking is *not* criticizing. Critical thinking is an analytical process that can help you think through a problem in an organized and efficient manner. Six steps are involved in critical thinking (Dressel and Mayhew, 1954). Thinking about these steps may help you when you work through the questions in your cases. In the beginning, it may help for you to write everything down on the Case Study Worksheet (Appendix B) as you learn the process of discovery. Here are the six steps with an explanation of what they mean.

1. Define the problem by asking the right questions: Exactly what is it you need to know? What is the question asking? Einstein once said that asking the right question was sometimes more important than having the right answer.
2. Select the information or data necessary to solve the problem or answer the question: First you have to ask whether all the necessary information is there. If not, how and where can you get the additional information? What other resources are available? This is one of the most difficult steps. In real clinical experiences, you rarely have all of the information, so you have to learn where you can get necessary data. For instance, patient and family interviews, nursing charting, the patient medical chart, laboratory data on your computer, your

observations, and your own physical assessment can help you identify important clues. Of course, information can rapidly become outdated. To make sure you are accessing the most current and accurate information, you will occasionally need to use a computer and the Internet to answer a question.

3. Recognize stated and unstated assumptions; that is, what do you think is or is not true? Sometimes answers or solutions seem obvious; just because something seems obvious doesn't mean it is correct. You may need to consider several possible answers or solutions. Consider all clues carefully and *don't dismiss a possibility too quickly*. Remember, *"You never find an answer you don't think of."*

4. Formulate and select relevant and/or promising hypotheses: Think of these as hunches. Try to think of as many possibilities as you can. Consider the pros and cons of each.

5. Draw valid conclusions: Consider all data; then determine what is relevant and what makes the most sense. Only then should you draw your conclusions.

6. Consider the soundness of your decisions: Rethink your conclusions and decisions in light of the whole case. What is the best answer/solution? What could go wrong? This requires considering many different angles. Be willing to revise the conclusions you made in step 5 if new information or clues crop up. In today's health care settings, decision making often requires balancing the well-being needs of the patient with financial limitations imposed by the reimbursement system (this includes Medicare, Medicaid, and insurance companies). In making decisions, you need to take all the relevant issues into account. Remember, you may be asked to explain why you rejected other options.

It may look as if this kind of thinking comes naturally to instructors and experienced nurses. You can be certain that even experienced professionals were once where you are now. (Sometimes they seem to forget that!) The rapid and sound decision making that is essential to good nursing requires years of practice. The practice of good clinical thinking leads to good thinking in clinical practice. This book will help you practice the important steps in making sound clinical judgments again and again, until the process starts to come naturally.

The practice of good clinical thinking leads to good thinking in clinical practice.

Rating Questions

The questions or problems related to cases in this book have been rated according to their level of complexity. Each category requires a more sophisticated level of thinking than the previous. Sometimes different types of questions or problems will be mixed together in the same case. The five categories are as follows.

1. **Knowledge**—This represents information, data, or facts and deals with questions like *Who? What? When? Where?* and *How much?*

2. **Comprehension**—This involves understanding the importance, significance, or meaning of specific information or facts.

3. **Application**—This involves understanding the information or facts and implementing or using them. Application also involves figuring out what—of all the information in a given setting—is important and appropriate to the problem and applying that information to a plan of action. Each setting contains a lot of information; some of it is not relevant. In some settings, certain information may even lead to false conclusions.

4. **Analysis**—This involves criticism and evaluation and requires taking a situation or problem apart to figure out what is going on (or going wrong). Analysis involves gaining knowledge, understanding the meaning or significance of that knowledge, and recognizing how it can best be applied. It also involves evaluating ("figuring out") what is wrong or anticipating what can go wrong. In finding out what is wrong, you will encounter one or more assumptions that may lead to false conclusions or something that you don't understand.

5. **Synthesis**—This is a more advanced kind of thinking that requires combining, arranging, incorporating, integrating, or coordinating what you know to arrive at a specific result. Synthesis is a creative process that involves pulling everything together. This type of thinking is characteristic of advanced clinicians. In a deeper sense, although the questions in these cases are not synthesis-type questions, your brain is constantly in "synthesis mode." Indeed, that's why case studies help develop your critical thinking skills—they help you learn to open new brain pathways in a way that memorization cannot.

The "How to" of Case Studies

When you begin each case, read through the whole story once, from start to finish, to get a general idea what it is about. Get out your Case Study Worksheet and write down things you had to look up. That way you won't have to look them up a second or third time. This is your "cheat sheet." This will help you move through the case smoothly and get more out of it. How much you have to look up will depend on where you are in your program, what you know, and how much experience you already have. Preparing cases will become easier as you advance in your program.

Acknowledgments

I would like to thank:

Our patients, who let us learn nursing by practicing on them.

Those nurses we saw in action and told ourselves, "Now *that's* a great nurse!"

The teachers who encouraged us to follow our convictions.

And to those who have bequeathed to us a nursing heritage of integrity, excellence, courage, and service.

To them I humbly acknowledge our gratitude and indebtedness.

This book would never have become a reality if not for the forbearance and help of the following individuals:

Kristin Geen, Acquisitions Editor

Lauren Lake, Senior Developmental Editor

And the consultants, for the creative work they shared and for their sharp eyes that picked up on errors. I thank you for your unflagging support.

I would like to offer a special tribute to the people who said, "It can't be done," "It'll never work," and "We've never done it that way," and thereby challenged us to prove them wrong.

B.A.P.

Contents

Contents

Contents

Contents

Cardiovascular Disorders

Case Study 1

Name _____ Class/Group _____ Date _____
Group Members _____
INSTRUCTIONS All questions apply to this case study. Your responses should be brief and to the point. When asked to provide several answers, list them in order of priority or significance. Do not assume information that is not provided. Please print or write clearly. If your response is not legible, it will be marked as ? and you will need to rewrite it.

Scenario

M.G., a "frequent flier," is admitted to the emergency department (ED) with a diagnosis of heart failure (HF). She was discharged from the hospital 10 days ago and comes in today stating, "I just had to come to the hospital today because I can't catch my breath and my legs are as big as tree trunks." After further questioning you learn she is strictly following the fluid and salt restriction ordered during her last hospital admission. She reports gaining 1 to 2 pounds every day since her discharge.

1. What error in teaching most likely occurred when M.G. was discharged 10 days ago?

CASE STUDY PROGRESS

You chart the medications M.G. brought with her: enalapril (Vasotec) 5 mg bid, digoxin 0.125 mg/day, rosiglitazone 4 mg, furosemide 40 mg/day, and potassium chloride 20 mEq/day. The admitting provider orders all the medications but changes the furosemide to 80 mg IV push (IVP) now, then 40 mg/day IVP.

2. What is the rationale for changing the method of administering furosemide?

3. You administer furosemide 80 mg IVP. Identify three parameters you would use to monitor the effectiveness of this medication.

4. What laboratory tests should be ordered for M.G. related to (R/T) the order for furosemide?

✳ **Note:** *Most HF admissions are R/T fluid volume overload. Patients who do not require intensive care monitoring can most often be treated initially with IVP diuretics, O$_2$, and angiotensin-converting enzyme (ACE) inhibitors.*

5. How do ACE inhibitors help in HF?

6. M.G.'s symptoms improve with IV diuretics. She is ordered back on oral furosemide once her weight loss is deemed adequate to achieve a euvolemic state. What will determine if the oral dose will be adequate to consider her for discharge?

7. M.G. is ready for discharge. What key management concepts should be taught to prevent relapse and another admission?

✳ **Hint:** *Use the mnemonic MAWDS.*

Case Study **2**

Name _____ Class/Group _____ Date _____

Group Members _____

INSTRUCTIONS All questions apply to this case study. Your responses should be brief and to the point. When asked to provide several answers, list them in order of priority or significance. Do not assume information that is not provided. Please print or write clearly. If your response is not legible, it will be marked as ? and you will need to rewrite it.

Scenario

M.P. is a lively 78-year-old African-American woman who comes to your clinic for a follow-up (F/U) visit. She was diagnosed (Dx) with hypertension (HTN) 2 months ago and was given a prescription for hydrochlorothiazide (HCTZ) 25 mg/day but stopped taking it because "it made me dizzy and I kept getting up during the night to empty my bladder." She comes to the clinic because her mother died of a cerebrovascular accident (CVA, stroke) at her age and she is afraid she will suffer the same fate. Vital signs (VS) during her initial visit were as follows: 160/102, 78, 16, 36.8°C. She is a lifetime non-smoker, nondrinker. Her father died of a myocardial infarction (MI) at 67 years of age. One brother is alive but has coronary artery disease (CAD), diabetes mellitus (DM), and HTN. Her sister is alive and well (A&W) at 62 years of age. Her basic metabolic panel (BMP) and fasting lipids were within normal limits (WNL).

1. After a 10-minute waiting period, you take M.P.'s blood pressure (BP) and get 156/96 mm Hg. According to the most recent Joint National Committee on Prevention, Detection, Evaluation, and Treatment of High Blood Pressure (JNC) Risk Stratification and Treatment Recommendations, what risk group is she in, and what stage of HTN does her BP represent?

CASE STUDY PROGRESS

She goes on to ask whether there is anything else she should do to help with her HTN. Remember, she is 5'4" and weighs 110 pounds. She has never smoked. Her glucose and lipid levels are within normal range.

2. Look up M.P.'s height and weight for her age on a body mass index (BMI) chart. Is she considered overweight? Why or why not? Explain which method you used to determine your answer and where you got your information.

   ❋**Hint:** *You can use any one of a number of charts or calculations.*

3. What nonpharmacologic lifestyle alteration measures might help someone like M.P. control her BP? List one and explain.

✳ **Note:** *Not everyone responds the same way to lifestyle modifications or medications. There is often a need for trial and error in establishing the best medication or combination of interventions to manage a health problem. Considerations include (1) how many and what specific side effects are experienced by the individual, (2) how acceptable those side effects are, (3) interactions with medications for other conditions or diseases, (4) cost of the medications, (5) whether the person responds favorably to the medication, and (6) difficulty in taking medications.*

4. When someone is taking HCTZ, what laboratory tests would you expect to be monitored? (List at least two.)

CASE STUDY PROGRESS
Because M.P.'s BP continues to be high, the internist decides to put her on another drug.

5. According to national guidelines, what is another recommended drug category for elderly nondiabetic individuals? Should this be used independently, with her current medication, or with another new drug?

CASE STUDY PROGRESS
The internist decreases her HCTZ to 12.5 mg and adds a prescription for lisinopril 10 mg (normal dose is 20 mg, but since this is an older woman, the rule is to start low, go slow). M.P. is instructed to return to the clinic to have her potassium checked in 1 week. She is also to monitor her BP at least twice a week and return for a medication management appointment in 1 month with her list of BP readings.

6. In doing your teaching, what side effects would you ask her to watch for and notify your office if she experiences?

7. It is sometimes difficult to remember whether you've taken your medication. What techniques might you teach M.P. to help her remember to take her medication each day? (Name at least two.)

CASE STUDY PROGRESS

M.P. returns in 1 month for her medication management appointment. She tells you she is feeling fine and does not have any side effects from her new medication. Her BP, checked twice a week at the senior center, ranges from 132 to 136/78 to 82 mm Hg.

8. You take M.P.'s BP and get 134/82 mm Hg. She asks whether these BP readings are OK. On what do you base your response?

9. List at least three important ways you might help her maintain her success.

CASE STUDY PROGRESS

M.P. comes in for a routine F/U visit 3 months later. She continues to do well on her daily BP drug regimen, with average BP readings of 130/78 mm Hg. She participates in a group walking program at the senior center. She admits she has not done as well with decreasing her salt intake. She tells you she recently was at a luncheon with her garden club and that most of those women take different BP pills than she does. She asks why their pills are different shapes and colors.

10. How can you explain the difference to M.P.?

Bonus Problem

The cost of medications is a critical issue for elderly individuals on a fixed income. To help you develop a sensitivity to the cost of prescriptions, have one person in your study group call to see whether there are generic versions of the medications M.P. is receiving and how much she would pay for a 30-day supply (don't have everybody call the pharmacy at once). Although not all generic drugs are "created equal" in terms of bioavailability (look this one up), see what is the least expensive option for M.P.

Bonus Problem

Remind M.P. that she should continue with her prescribed medications and not make any alterations. Especially emphasize the need to talk with you or the physician before she starts taking any "natural" or herbal remedies, over-the-counter (OTC) remedies for cold or flu, or nutritional supplements. Name one herbal remedy or natural product that could elevate her BP.

Case Study **3**

Scenario

You are a nurse at a freestanding cardiac prevention and rehabilitation center. Your new patient in risk-factor modification is B.J., a 37-year-old traveling salesman, who is married and has 3 children. During a recent evaluation for chest pain, he underwent a cardiac catheterization procedure that showed moderate single-vessel disease with a 50% stenosis in the mid right coronary artery (RCA). He was given a prescription for sublingual (SL) nitroglycerin (NTG), told how to use it, and referred to your cardiac rehabilitation program for sessions 3 days a week. B.J.'s wife comes along to help him with healthy lifestyle changes. You take the following nursing history: B.J.'s father died of sudden cardiac death at age 42, and his mother (still living) had a quadruple coronary artery bypass graft (CABG ×4) at age 52; his hypertension (HTN) is controlled by taking metoprolol 25 mg q12h, which was also prescribed for his coronary disease, as well as by taking acetylsalicylic acid (ASA, aspirin) 325 mg/day PO; he has averaged 1.5 packs of cigarettes per day (PPD) for 20 years; an "occasional" beer ("a 6-pack every weekend with the football game"*); and a dietary history of fried and fast foods. His current weight is 235 pounds at 5'8"; he has a waist circumference of 48 inches. His vital signs (VS) are 138/88, 82, 18, and 98.4° F.

> ✳ **Note:** *Be alert to the fact that many individuals tend to underreport their alcohol and drug consumption. Clearly mark patient reports by using quotes to indicate subjective source of information.*

1. Calculate B.J.'s smoking history in terms of pack–years.

2. List three nonmodifiable risk factors for coronary artery disease (CAD).

3. List six modifiable risk factors for CAD.

4. Underline each of the responses in questions 2 and 3 that represent B.J.'s personal CAD risk factors.

5. You would like to know more about B.J.'s hyperlipidemia. What four common laboratory values do you need to know?

CASE STUDY PROGRESS

B.J. laughingly tells you he believes in the 5 all-American food groups: salt, sugar, fat, chocolate, and caffeine.

6. Identify health-related problems in this case description; the problem that is potentially life threatening should be listed first.

7. Of all his behaviors, which one is the most significant in promoting cardiac disease?

8. What is the highest priority problem that you need to address with B.J.? Identify the teaching strategy you would use with him.
   ✻**Hint:** *What you think is the most important may not be what he considers the most important, or the one he is willing to work on.*

✳ **9.** What is the second problem you would work with B.J. to change? Identify an appropriate strategy to resolve the problem.

✳ **Note:** *Whenever B.J. and his wife decide to attack dietary changes, try to get a referral to a registered dietitian (RD), who can work with them to develop strategies for long-term nutritional goals to decrease HTN and serum lipids. Many states require dietitians to be licensed the same way nurses are registered. Check to make certain that nutritional counseling for a person with specific disease states is not exceeding the nursing standard of practice for your state.*

10. B.J.'s wife takes you aside and tells you, "I'm so worried for B. I grew up in a really dysfunctional family where there was a lot of violence. B. has been so good to the kids and me. I'm so worried I'll lose him that I have nightmares about his heart stopping. I find myself suddenly awakening at night just to see if he's breathing." How are you going to respond?

✳ **Note:** *Nightmares about losing a loved one to heart disease are not rare, especially during the time of diagnosis or disease-related crisis. However, a background of childhood violence can have deep roots and often requires special help. Clearly this woman is in distress. Depending on her willingness at this time, it would be good for her to talk with a therapist. If she doesn't think she needs it, try suggesting that it might be good for B.J. and the kids and that it would help her relax and be more responsive to them. At the appropriate point, it would be important for her to be able to share with her husband how she feels. From her description, this sleep disturbance is an unhealthy situation that should be addressed. If she refuses, keep an open relationship; it is important that she keep talking to someone about her fear.*

CASE STUDY PROGRESS
Six weeks after you start working with B.J., he admits that he has been under a lot of stress. He rubs his chest and says, "It feels really heavy on my chest right now." You feel his pulse and note that his skin is slightly diaphoretic, and that he is agitated and appears to be anxious.

11. What are you going to do to obtain additional information?

12. B.J. continues to feel symptomatic. Now what are you going to do?

Case Study **4**

Name _____ Class/Group _____ Date _____
Group Members _____
INSTRUCTIONS All questions apply to this case study. Your responses should be brief and to the point. When asked to provide several answers, list them in order of priority or significance. Do not assume information that is not provided. Please print or write clearly. If your response is not legible, it will be marked as ? and you will need to rewrite it.

Scenario

S.P. is a 68-year-old (yo) retired painter who is experiencing right leg calf pain. The pain began approximately 2 years ago but has become significantly worse in the past 4 months. The pain is precipitated by exercise and is relieved with rest. Two years ago S.P. could walk 2 city blocks before having to stop due to leg pain. Today he can barely walk across the kitchen. S.P. has smoked 2 to 3 packs of cigarettes per day (PPD) for the past 45 years. He has a history of coronary artery disease (CAD), hypertension (HTN), peripheral vascular disease (PVD), and osteoarthritis. Surgical history includes quadruple coronary artery bypass graft (CABG ×4) 3 years ago. He has had no further symptoms of cardiopulmonary disease since that time despite the fact that he has not been compliant with the exercise regimen his cardiologist prescribed, continues to eat anything he wants, and continues to smoke 2 to 3 PPD. Other surgical history includes open reduction internal fixation (ORIF) of the right femoral fracture 20 years ago.

In clinic today, S.P.'s weight is 261 pounds; height is 5'10"; vital signs (VS) are 163/91, 82, 16, afebrile. His fasting lipids are cholesterol 239 mg/dl, triglyceride 150 mg/dl, HDL 28 mg/dl, LDL 181 mg/dl. Medications include lisinopril 20 mg/day, metoprolol 25 mg bid, aspirin 325 mg/day, simvastatin 40 mg/day.

1. S.P. is in clinic today for a routine semiannual follow-up (F/U) appointment with his primary care provider. You are taking his blood pressure (BP) and he tells you that, besides the calf pain, he is experiencing right hip pain that gets worse with exercise, doesn't go away promptly with rest, some days is worse than others, and is not affected by resting position. What are the likely sources of his calf pain and his hip pain?

2. S.P. has several risk factors for claudication. From his history, list two risk factors and explain why they are risk factors.

3. You decide to look at S.P.'s lower extremities. What signs would you expect to find with intermittent claudication? Identify four findings.

4. Where would you expect S.P. to complain of pain if he had superficial femoral artery stenosis? Popliteal stenosis?

CASE STUDY PROGRESS

His primary care provider has seen S.P. and wants you to schedule the patient for an ankle-brachial index (ABI) test to determine the presence of arterial blood flow obstruction. You confirm the time and date of the procedure and then call S.P. at home.

5. What will you tell S.P. to do to prepare for the tests?

CASE STUDY PROGRESS

S.P.'s ABI results showed 0.33 right (R) leg and 0.59 left (L) leg. These results indicate he has severe arterial obstruction in his right leg and moderate obstruction in his left leg.

6. You counsel S.P. on risk factor modification. What would you address and why?

7. In addition to risk factor modification, what other measures to improve tissue perfusion or prevent skin damage should you recommend to S.P.?

8. S.P. tells you his neighbor told him to keep his legs elevated higher than his heart and ask for compression stockings to keep swelling in his legs down. How should you respond?

9. S.P. recently got hit on the right shin with a softball and now complains of constant right lower extremity pain. What should you be concerned about?

CASE STUDY PROGRESS

You caution S.P. to avoid repeated injury to his already compromised leg. He assures you he doesn't want to lose his leg and will be more careful in the future.

Case Study **5**

Scenario

You are the nurse working in an anticoagulation clinic. K.N. is a patient who has a longstanding irregularly irregular heartbeat (atrial fibrillation, or A-fib) for which he takes the oral anticoagulant warfarin (Coumadin). Recently, K.N. had his mitral heart valve replaced with a mechanical valve. You know that there are different PT/INR (prothrombin time/International Normalized Ratio) goal recommendations based on the indication for anticoagulation. (NOTE: PT has now been replaced by or is reported, in most cases, with INR [International Normalized Ratio], an international value that allows for laboratory standardization. PTT is more properly written aPTT [activated partial thromboplastin time]; however, PTT is still in common clinical use.) A-fib carries an INR therapeutic goal range of 2.0 to 3.0. Mechanical valves in the mitral position are considered at greater thromboembolic risk than the aortic site. Therefore K.N. will need his PT/INR to be kept at the higher goal range of 2.5 to 3.5.

K.N. calls your anticoagulation clinic to report a nosebleed that is hard to stop. He asks to come into the office to check his clotting time. When you get the results, his INR is critical at 7.2. The provider has asked you to inform the patient that the level is too high.

1. What should you tell K.N.?

✳ **Note:** *INR is a mathematic calculation to convert PT to an internationally reported ratio. The INR number is not followed by any unit of measure.*

CASE STUDY PROGRESS

The provider does a brief focused history and physical examination, orders additional lab tests, and determines that there are no signs of bleeding. The provider discovers that K.N. recently went to the local emergency department (ED) for a sinus infection and had received a prescription for sulfamethoxazole and trimethoprim (Septra), an antibiotic that has a significant interaction with warfarin.

2. What should K.N. have done to prevent this problem?

3. The provider gives K.N. a low dose of vitamin K orally, asks him to hold his warfarin dose that evening, and asks him to come back tomorrow for another PT/INR blood draw. What should you tell K.N. about vitamin K?

4. You want to make certain K.N. knows what "hold the next dose" means. What should you tell him?

5. K.N. asks you why his PT/INR has to be checked so soon. How should you respond?

6. K.N.'s INR the next day is 3.7. Although the INR is a little elevated, the provider made no further medication changes. K.N. is instructed to finish the remaining 2 days of antibiotics and return again in 7 days to have another PT/INR drawn. Why should the INR be checked again so soon instead of the usual monthly follow-up (F/U)?

7. K.N. grumbles about all the lab tests but agrees to follow through. The next INR is 2.8. What patient education needs to be stressed at this visit? Identify two education needs.

8. Six months later, K.N. informs you that he is going to have a knee replacement next month. What should you do with this information?

CASE STUDY PROGRESS

You know that sometimes the only needed action is to stop the warfarin several days before the surgery. Other times the provider initiates "bridging therapy," or stops the warfarin and provides anticoagulation protection by initiating unfractionated heparin or low-molecular-weight heparin. After reviewing all his anticoagulation information, the provider decides that K.N. should be on enoxaparin (Lovenox) before surgery.

9. How should you explain the importance of enoxaparin to K.N.?

CASE STUDY PROGRESS

Your next patient has a history of taking his medication sporadically and doesn't show up for his PT/INR testing on a regular basis. His noncompliance is not due to financial problems or cognitive impairment.

10. What content areas should you address during this patient encounter?

CASE STUDY PROGRESS

Your third patient is returning for an F/U visit. At the last visit you found a new irregularly irregular heart rate on auscultation. An ECG confirmed A-fib. His Holter monitor, chest x-ray (CXR), CBC, thyroid-stimulating hormone (TSH), and chem 14 (chemistry panel) have been completed, and the patient returns today to discuss the results and needs to be informed that the provider has scheduled the patient for cardioversion.

11. What educational needs should you address today?

Case Study **6**

Scenario

You are working in the internal medicine clinic of a large teaching hospital. Today your first patient is 70-year-old J.M., a man who has been coming to the clinic for several years for management of coronary artery disease (CAD), hypertension (HTN), and anemia. A cardiac catheterization done a year ago showed 50% stenosis of the circumflex coronary artery. He has had episodes of dizziness for the past 6 months and orthostatic hypotension, shoulder discomfort, and decreased exercise tolerance for the past 2 months. On his last clinic visit 3 weeks ago, a chest x-ray (CXR) showed cardiomegaly and a 12-lead ECG showed left bundle branch block (LBBB). Results of chemistries (blood studies) drawn at this time were as follows: Na 136 mmol/L, K 5.2 mmol/L, BUN 15 mg/dl, creatinine 1.8 mg/dl, glucose 82 mg/dl, Cl 95 mmol/L, CBC: WBC 4.4 thou/cmm, Hgb 10.5 g/dl, Hct 31.4%, and platelets 229 thou/cmm. (NOTE: The former *mm*^{3} for cubic millimeters is currently written *Thou* or *thou/cmm*.) This morning his daughter brought him to the clinic because he has had increased fatigue, significant swelling of his ankles, and shortness of breath (SOB) for the past 2 days. His vital signs (VS) are 142/83, 105, 18, and 97.9°F.

1. Knowing his history and seeing his condition this morning, what further questions are you going to ask J.M. and his daughter?

CASE STUDY PROGRESS

J.M. tells you he becomes exhausted and has SOB climbing the stairs to his bedroom and has to lie down and rest ("put my feet up") at least an hour twice a day. He has been sleeping on 2 pillows for the past 2 weeks. He has not salted his food since the physician told him not to because of his high blood pressure (BP), but he admits having had ham and a whole bag of salted peanuts 3 days ago. He denies having palpitations but has had a constant, irritating, nonproductive cough lately.

2. You think it likely that J.M. has heart failure (HF). From his history, what do you identify as probable causes for his HF?

3. You are now ready to do your physical assessment. List at least nine things you would assess to confirm or disconfirm your suspicion about the HF. Also indicate with an "L" or an "R" whether the sign is due to left-sided or right-sided HF, or both.

4. The physician confirms your suspicion that J.M. is experiencing symptoms of HF. What classes of medications might the physician prescribe?

5. This is J.M.'s first episode of significant HF. Before he leaves the clinic, you want to teach him about lifestyle modifications he can make and monitoring techniques he can use to prevent or minimize future problems. List five suggestions you might make and the rationale for each.

6. You tell J.M. the combination of high-sodium foods he had during the past several days may have caused his present episode of HF. He looks surprised. J.M. says, "But I didn't add any salt to them!" To what health care professional could J.M. be referred to help him understand how to prevent future crises? State your rationale.

7. J.M. receives a prescription for furosemide with a potassium (K) supplement. He wrinkles his nose at the suggestion of K and tells you he "hates those horse pills." He tells you a friend of his said he could eat bananas instead. He says he would rather eat a banana every day than take one of those pills. How will you respond?

8. It's winter and today's temperature is 15° F. J.M. tells you he's been getting cold feet lately. This has never bothered him before. What would you suggest as comfort and safety measures?

9. Researchers sometimes call the legs "the second heart." In view of this statement and J.M.'s cardiac history, explain why "walking would be better than standing" for his circulation.

Case Study **7**

Scenario

It is midmorning on the cardiac unit where you work, and you are getting a new patient. G.P. is a 60-year-old retired businessman, who is married and has 3 grown children. As you take his health history, he tells you that he began feeling changes in his heart rhythm about 10 days ago. He has hypertension (HTN) and a 5-year history of angina pectoris. During the past week he has had frequent episodes of mid-chest discomfort. The chest pain has awakened him from sleep but does respond to nitroglycerin (NTG), which he has taken sublingually (SL) about 8 to 10 times over the past week. During the week he has also experienced increased fatigue. He states, "I just feel crappy all the time anymore." A cardiac catheterization done several years ago revealed 50% stenosis of the right coronary artery (RCA) and 50% stenosis of the left anterior descending (LAD) coronary artery. He tells you that both his mother and father had coronary artery disease (CAD). He is taking amlodipine, metoprolol, atorvastatin (Lipitor), and baby aspirin 81 mg/day.

1. What other information are you going to ask about his episodes of chest pain?

2. What are common sites for radiation of ischemic cardiac pain?

✳ **Note:** *Patients will tell you what they think you want to hear, so be careful how you ask your questions.*

3. You know that G.P. has atherosclerosis of the coronary arteries, but he has not told you about his risk factors. You need to know his risk factors for CAD in order to plan teaching for lifestyle modifications. What will you ask him about?

4. Although he has been taking SL NTG for a long time, you want to be certain he is using it correctly. What information would you need to make certain he understands the side effects, use, and storage of SL NTG?

CASE STUDY PROGRESS
When you first admitted G.P., you placed him on telemetry and observed he was in atrial fibrillation (A-fib) converting frequently to atrial flutter with a 4:1 block. His vital signs (VS) and all of his lab tests were within normal range, including troponin and creatinine phosphokinase (CK) levels; potassium (K) was 4.7 mmol/L. He spontaneously converted with medication (diltiazem) from A-fib/atrial flutter to tachycardia/bradycardia syndrome with long sinus pauses that caused lightheadedness and hypotension.

5. What risks does the new rhythm pose for G.P.?

CASE STUDY PROGRESS

Because G.P.'s dysrhythmia is causing unacceptable symptoms, he is taken to surgery and a permanent DDI pacemaker is placed and set at a rate of 70 beats/min.

6. What does the code "DDI" mean?

7. The pacemaker insertion surgery places G.P. at risk for several serious complications. List three potential problems that you will monitor for as you care for him.

8. G.P. will need some education regarding his new pacemaker. What information will you give him before he leaves the hospital?

✳ **Note:** *Information about the MedicAlert emergency identification system can be obtained by calling (800) 432-5378.*

9. G.P.'s wife approaches you and anxiously inquires, "My neighbor saw this science fiction movie about this guy who got a pacemaker and then he couldn't die. Is that for real?" How are you going to respond to her?

10. G.P. and his wife tell you they have heard that people with pacemakers can have their hearts stop because of theft and security sensors in stores and airports. Where can you help them find more information?

CASE STUDY PROGRESS

After discharge, G.P. is referred to a cardiac prevention and rehabilitation center to start an exercise program. He will be exercise tested, and an individualized exercise prescription will be developed for him based on the exercise test.

11. What information will be obtained from the graded exercise (stress) test (GXT), and what is included in an exercise prescription?

Case Study **8**

Scenario

You are assigned to care for L.J., a 70-year-old retired bus driver who has just been admitted to your medical floor with right leg deep vein thrombosis (DVT). L.J. has a 48-pack-year smoking history, although he states he quit 2 years ago. He has had pneumonia several times and frequent episodes of atrial fibrillation (A-fib). He has had 2 previous episodes of DVT and was diagnosed with rheumatoid arthritis 3 years ago. Two months ago he began experiencing shortness of breath (SOB) on exertion and noticed swelling of his right foreleg (lower leg) that became progressively worse until it extended up to his groin. His wife brought him to the hospital when he complained of (C/O) increasingly severe pain in his leg. When a Doppler study indicated a probable thrombus of the external iliac vein extending distally to the lower leg, he was admitted for bed rest and to initiate heparin therapy. Significant admission laboratory values are PT 12.4 sec, INR 1.11, PTT 25 sec, Hgb 13.3 g/dl, Hct 38.9%, and cholesterol 206 mg/dl. Basic metabolic panel (BMP) is normal.

1. Look up the external iliac vein in your anatomy book. List six risk factors for DVT.

2. Identify at least five problems from L.J.'s history that represent his personal risk factors.

3. Something is missing from the scenario. Based on his history, L.J. should have been taking an important medication. What is it, and why should he be taking it?

✳ **4.** Keeping in mind L.J.'s health history and admitting diagnosis, what are the most important assessments you should make during your physical examination and assessment?

5. What is the most serious complication of DVT?

CASE STUDY PROGRESS

Your assessment of L.J. reveals bibasilar crackles with moist cough; normal heart sounds; blood pressure (BP) 138/88 mm Hg; pulse 104 beats/min; 3+ pitting edema right lower extremity; mild erythema of right foot and calf; and severe right calf pain. He is awake, alert, and oriented (AAO) but a little restless. He denies having SOB and chest pain.

6. List at least eight assessment findings you should monitor closely for development of the complication identified in question 5.

✳ **Note:** *If a pulmonary embolism is massive, the signs and symptoms (S/S) are more like those of myocardial infarction (MI): crushing, substernal chest pain; marked respiratory distress; feeling of impending doom; rapid, shallow breathing; bloody sputum; severe SOB; dysrhythmias; and shock.*

CASE STUDY PROGRESS

L.J. is placed on 72-hour BR (bed rest) with BRP (bathroom privileges) and given acetaminophen (Tylenol) for pain.

7. Enoxaparin 70 mg (0.7 ml) is prescribed for systemic anticoagulation. L.J. is 5′6″ and weighs 156 pounds. What kind of drug is enoxaparin? Is this dose appropriate? How would it be administered?

8. What instructions will you give L.J. about his activity?

9. What pertinent laboratory values or test results would you expect the physician to order and you to monitor?

10. You identify pain as a key issue in the care of L.J. List four interventions you would choose for L.J. to address his pain.

11. (Optional) This is a copy of one of the ECGs taken from L.J. Identify rate, rhythm, QRS after each P, PR interval, and QRS interval. Are sinus and ventricular rhythm the same? Name this rhythm.

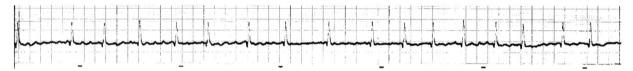

CASE STUDY PROGRESS

A week has passed. L.J. responded to heparin therapy, was started on warfarin therapy, and is being discharged home with home care follow-up (F/U). "Good," he says, "just in time to fly out West for my grandson's wedding." His wife, who has come to pick him up, rolls her eyes and looks at the ceiling. You almost drop the discharge papers in disbelief. (And you thought you did such a good job of discharge teaching!)

12. What are you going to tell him?

CASE STUDY PROGRESS

L.J. listens to you, and Mrs. J. is quite relieved. (She has been telling her friends about this "wonderful nurse who talked some sense into my husband.") L.J.'s son arranges to videotape the wedding cere-mony, and guests at the reception record special greetings for him. It's been 2 weeks, and he seems quite pleased. He watches the tape daily and points out his favorite parts to the home care nurse every time she visits.

Case Study **9**

Name _____ Class/Group_____ Date _____
Group Members _____

INSTRUCTIONS All questions apply to this case study. Your responses should be brief and to the point. When asked to provide several answers, list them in order of priority or significance. Do not assume information that is not provided. Please print or write clearly. If your response is not legible, it will be marked as ? and you will need to rewrite it.

Scenario

A.H. is a 70-year-old retired construction worker who has experienced lumbosacral pain, nausea, and upset stomach for the past 6 months. He has a history of heart failure (HF), deep visceral pain, dyspnea, hypertension (HTN), sleep apnea, and depression. A.H. has just been admitted to the hospital for surgical repair of a 6.2-cm abdominal aortic aneurysm (AAA) that is now causing him constant pain. On arrival on your floor, his vital signs (VS) are 109/81, 61, 16, and 98.3° F. When you perform your assessment, you find that his apical heart rhythm is regular and his peripheral pulses are strong. His lungs are clear, and he is awake, alert, and oriented (AAO). There are no abnormal physical findings; however, he hasn't had a bowel movement for 3 days. His electrolytes and other blood chemistries and clotting studies are within normal range, but his hematocrit (Hct) is 30.1% and hemoglobin (Hgb) is 9 g/dl.

A.H. has been depressed since the death of his wife 9 years ago. He has no children. He is 6'2" tall and weighs 160 pounds. His chronic medical problems have been managed over the years by medications: benazepril 40 mg/day PO, fluoxetine 40 mg/day PO, furosemide 40 mg/day PO, trazodone 50 mg PO qhs, KCl 20 mEq PO bid, and lovastatin 40 mg PO with the evening meal.

1. A.H. has several common risk factors for AAA, which are evident from his health history. Identify and explain three factors.

CASE STUDY PROGRESS

While A.H. awaits his surgery, it is important that you monitor him carefully for decrease in tissue perfusion.

2. Identify five things you would assess for, and state your rationale for each.

3. What is the most serious, life-threatening complication of AAA, and why?

4. What single problem mentioned in the first paragraph of this case study presents a risk for AAA rupture? Why?

✳ **Note:** *Monitoring urinary output is critical in evaluating shock or for postsurvival problems.*

5. What is the minimal acceptable urinary output per hour?

CASE STUDY PROGRESS

The resection of A.H.'s aneurysm was successful, but for the first 3 postoperative days he was delirious and required one-to-one nursing care and soft restraints before he became coherent and oriented again. He was still somewhat confused when he was transferred back to your floor.

6. What assessments should be made specific to his postoperative care?

7. List five problems that should be high priorities in A.H.'s postoperative care.

8. Postoperative care of the patient undergoing aneurysmectomy includes preservation of the graft, preservation of tissue perfusion, and prevention of infection. List three interventions that would address these issues, and explain the rationale for each.

CASE STUDY PROGRESS
When A.H. is being prepared for discharge, you talk to him about health promotion and lifestyle change issues that are pertinent to his health problems.

9. Identify four health-related issues you might appropriately address with him and what you would teach in each area.

10. A.H. will be receiving follow-up (F/U) visits from the home health care nurse to change his dressing and evaluate his incision. What can you discuss with A.H. before discharge that will help him understand what the nurse will be doing?

11. What link could there be between A.H.'s diet and his depression?

✢ **Note:** *Make certain there is a physician's order for medical nutrition therapy (MNT) for A.H. He is going to need a lot of help maintaining a healthy diet specific to his needs. RDs are often aware of community resources that could help someone like A.H.*

Case Study **10**

Scenario

R.K. is an 85-year-old woman who lives with her husband, who is 87. Two nights before her admission
to your cardiac unit, she awoke with heavy substernal pressure accompanied by epigastric distress.
The pain was reduced somewhat when she rolled onto her side but did not completely subside for
about 6 hours. The next night she experienced the same chest pressure. The following morning, R.K.'s
husband took her to the physician, and she was subsequently hospitalized to rule out myocardial
infarction (R/O MI). Labs were drawn in the emergency department (ED). She was started on oxygen
(O_2) at 2 L via nasal cannula (NC) and given nonenteric-coated aspirin 325 mg to be chewed and swal-
lowed. An IV was started.

You obtain the following information from your history and physical examination: R.K. has no history
of smoking or alcohol use, and she has been in good general health with the exception of osteoarthritis
of her hands and knees and some osteoarthritis of the spine. Her only medications are ranitidine, ibuprofen for bone and joint pain, and "herbs." Her admission vital signs (VS) are 132/84, 88, 18, and
37.2°C. Her weight is 52 kg and height is 163 cm. Moderate edema of both ankles is present, but
capillary refill is brisk and peripheral pulses are 1+. You hear a soft systolic murmur. You place her on
telemetry, which shows frequent premature atrial contractions (PACs) but no ventricular ectopy. She
denies any discomfort at present.

1. Give at least two reasons an IV would be inserted. What kind of IV fluid would you
   expect to be running and at what rate? (This question requires a series of mental steps.
   First, you need to gather your facts, and then you need to figure out what they mean. You
   need to analyze this context, and then decide what is appropriate to use.)

2. Why is "nonenteric–coated" aspirin specified? What would be a contraindication to
   administering aspirin?

3. R.K. becomes fatigued during the admission process, and you decide to let her sleep. When she awakens, what additional history and physical information should you obtain related to (R/T) her admitting diagnosis?

4. List seven laboratory or diagnostic tests you would expect were drawn or conducted in the ED; suggest what each may contribute.

5. What other source, besides cardiac ischemia, may be responsible for her chest and abdominal discomfort? (Specify.)

6. Define the concept *differential diagnosis*.

7. Explain how the concept of differential diagnosis applies to R.K.'s symptoms.

8. Florence Nightingale frequently emphasized the value of good observation skills in nurses. Explain how a good nursing assessment can contribute to understanding the cause of R.K.'s symptoms.

9. Abnormalities on R.K.'s 12-lead ECG were reported as "slight left–axis deviation." Serial CK tests are 27 units/ml, 24 units/ml, 26 units/ml; troponin is less than 0.03 ng/ml. A series of tests R/O a noncardiac cause for her chest pain. On the basis of the information presented so far, do you believe she had an MI? What is your rationale?

10. While you care for R.K., you carefully observe her. Identify two possible complications of coronary artery disease (CAD) and the signs and symptoms (S/S) associated with each.

11. R.K. rings her call bell. When you arrive, she has her hand placed over her heart and tells you she is "having that heavy feeling again." She is not diaphoretic or nauseated but states she is short of breath (SOB). What can you do to make her more comfortable?

✳ **Note:** *Laboratory tests can be reported in terms of different values. Always read laboratory reports carefully to be sure which units are used in your institution.*

CASE STUDY PROGRESS

R.K.'s husband is upset. He tells you they have been married for 62 years and he doesn't know what he would do without his wife. One way to help people deal with their anxieties is to help them focus on concrete issues.

12. What information would be useful to get from him? What other health care professional may be able to help with some of these issues?

Case Study **11**

Name _____ **Class/Group** _____ **Date** _____

Group Members _____

INSTRUCTIONS All questions apply to this case study. Your responses should be brief and to the point. When asked to provide several answers, list them in order of priority or significance. Do not assume information that is not provided. Please print or write clearly. If your response is not legible, it will be marked as ? and you will need to rewrite it.

Scenario

The time is 1900 hours. You are working in a small, rural hospital. It has been snowing heavily all day, and the medical helicopters at the large regional medical center, 4 hours away by car (in good weather), have been grounded by the weather until morning. The roads are barely passable. W.R., a 48-year-old construction worker with a 36-pack-year smoking history, is admitted to your floor with a diagnosis of rule out myocardial infarction (R/O MI). He has significant male-pattern obesity ("beer belly," large waist circumference) and a barrel chest, and he reports a dietary history of high-fat food. His wife brought him to the emergency department (ED) after he complained of (C/O) unrelieved "indigestion." His admission vital signs (VS) were 202/124, 96, 18, and 98.2° F. W.R. was put on oxygen (O_2) by nasal cannula (NC) titrated to maintain Sao_2 (arterial oxygen saturation) over 90%, and an IV of nitroglycerin (NTG) was started in the ED. He was also given aspirin 325 mg and was admitted to Dr. A.'s service. There are plans to transfer him by helicopter to the regional medical center for a cardiac catheterization in the morning when the weather clears. Meanwhile you have to deal with limited laboratory and pharmacy resources. The minute W.R. comes through the door of your unit, he announces he's just fine in a loud and angry voice and demands a cigarette.

1. From the perspective of basic human needs, what is the first priority in his care?

2. Are these VS reasonable for a man his age? If not, which one(s) concern(s) you? Explain why or why not.

3. Identify five priority problems associated with the care of a patient like W.R.

4. Which of the following laboratory tests might be ordered to investigate W.R.'s condition? If the order is appropriate, place an "A" in the space provided. If inappropriate, mark with an "I," and provide rationales for your decisions.
   ___ 1. CBC
   ___ 2. EEG in the morning
   ___ 3. Chem 7 (electrolytes)
   ___ 4. PT/PTT
   ___ 5. Bilirubin every morning
   ___ 6. Urinalysis (UA)
   ___ 7. STAT 12-lead ECG
   ___ 8. Type and crossmatch (T&C) for 4 units packed RBCs (PRBCs)

5. What significant lab tests are missing from the previous list?

6. How are you going to respond to W.R.'s angry demands for a cigarette? He also demands something for his "heartburn." How will you respond?

CASE STUDY PROGRESS

You phone Dr. A.'s partner, who is "on call." She prescribes morphine sulfate 4 to 10 mg IV push (IVP) q1h prn for pain (burning, pressure, angina).

7. Explain two reasons for this order.

8. What special precautions should you follow when administering morphine sulfate IVP?

9. Angina is not always experienced as "pain" (as many people understand pain). How would you describe symptoms you want him to warn you about? Why is this important?

10. What safety measures or instructions would you give W.R. before you leave his room?

11. One of the housekeeping staff asks you, "If the poor guy can't smoke, why can't you give him one of those nicotine patches?" How will you respond?

12. If the patch were to be used later to help him quit smoking, how would it be dosed for him?

13. Before leaving for the night, Mrs. R. approaches you and asks, "Did my husband have a heart attack? I'm really scared. His father died of one when he was 51." How are you going to respond to her question?

14. When you come into W.R.'s room at 2200 hours to answer his call light, you see he is holding his left arm and C/O aching in his left shoulder and arm. What information are you going to gather? What questions will you ask him?

15. Based on your assessment findings, you decide to call the physician. What information are you going to report to the physician, and why?

CASE STUDY PROGRESS

In the morning W.R. is transferred by chopper to the medical center, and a cardiac catheterization is performed. It is determined that W.R. has coronary artery disease (CAD). The cardiologist suggests it would be best to treat him medically for now, with follow-up (F/U) counseling on risk factor modification, especially smoking cessation. He is discharged with a referral for an F/U visit to his local internist in 1 week.

16. What does it mean to treat him "medically" (conservatively)? What other approaches may be used to treat CAD?

17. What personality characteristic do you observe in W.R. that places him at high risk for CAD?

Case Study **12**

Name _____ Class/Group _____ Date _____
Group Members _____
INSTRUCTIONS All questions apply to this case study. Your responses should be brief and to the point. When asked to provide several answers, list them in order of priority or significance. Do not assume information that is not provided. Please print or write clearly. If your response is not legible, it will be marked as ? and you will need to rewrite it.

Scenario

You are working at the local cardiac rehabilitation center, and R.M. is walking around the track. He summons you and asks if you could help him understand his recent lab report. He admits to being confused by the overwhelming data on the test and doesn't understand how the results relate to his recent heart attack and need for a stent. You take a moment to locate his lab reports and review his history. Below are the findings.

R.M. is an active 61-year-old man who works full time for the postal service. He walks 3 miles every other day and admits he doesn't eat a "perfect diet." He enjoys 2 or 3 beers q noc (every night), he uses stick margarine, eats red meat 2 or 3 times per week, and is a self-professed "sweet eater." His cardiac history includes a recent inferior myocardial infarction (MI) and a heart catheterization revealing 3-vessel disease: in the left anterior descending (LAD) coronary artery, a proximal 60% lesion; in the right coronary artery (RCA), proximal 100% occlusion with thrombus; and a circumflex with 40% to 60% diffuse ectatic lesions. A stent was deployed to the RCA and reduced the lesion to 0% residual stenosis. He has had no need for nitroglycerin (NTG). He was discharged on aspirin 325 mg, clopidogrel (Plavix) 75 mg, atorvastatin (Lipitor) 10 mg, Foltx (folic acid, pyridoxine, and vitamin B_{12}) with food, and ramipril (Altace) 10 mg/day. Six weeks after his MI and stent deployment, he had a fasting advanced lipid profile. The results were total cholesterol 188 mg/dl, HDL 34 mg/dl, triglycerides 176 mg/dl, LDL 98 mg/dl, pattern B LDL typing at 19 nm, homocysteine 18 mg/dl, high-sensitivity C-reactive protein (HS CRP) 12 mg/dl, fasting blood glucose (FBG) 101 mg/dl, thyroid-stimulating hormone (TSH) 1.04 mg/dl.

1. Given the information above, what questions are important to ask R.M.?

2. When you start to discuss R.M.'s laboratory values with him, he is pleased that his total cholesterol is less than 200 mg/dl and that his low-density lipoprotein (LDL) is less than 100 mg/dl. He thinks he needs no further alteration in his lipid values. What do you tell him about his triglycerides and pattern B type?

3. R.M.'s physician adds niacin, folic acid, B_{12}, B_6, and omega-3 fatty acids to his list of medications. How do atorvastatin and the new medications affect lipids?

4. What treatment options are known to decrease CRP?

✳ **Note:** *All these treatments are thought to decrease inflammatory response in the arterial walls and endothelium. Many of these options should be used for primary prevention as well. They will reduce the number of cardiovascular events.*

5. HS CRP is an indicator of:

6. Identify the most common side effect of niacin and statins.

7. Elevated homocysteine can be a factor in what type of vascular complication?

8. Name one food or other substance that will increase the homocysteine level.

CASE STUDY PROGRESS

You enter R.M.'s room and hear the physician say, "There are many options to change the metabolic makeup of your small dense LDL and increased homocysteine. You need to continue modifying your diet and exercise to enhance your medication regimen." The physician asks R.M. if he has any questions, and the patient responds, "No."

9. After the physician leaves the room, R.M. tells you he really didn't understand what the physician said. Explain the necessary lifestyle changes to R.M.

10. A normal homocysteine level is:

Case Study **13**

Name _____ Class/Group _____ Date _____
Group Members _____
INSTRUCTIONS All questions apply to this case study. Your responses should be brief and to the point. When asked
to provide several answers, list them in order of priority or significance. Do not assume information that is not provided.
Please print or write clearly. If your response is not legible, it will be marked as ? and you will need to rewrite it.

Scenario

Your patient, 58-year-old K.Z., has a significant cardiac history. He has longstanding coronary artery disease (CAD) with occasional episodes of heart failure (HF). One year ago he had an anterior wall myocardial infarction (MI). In addition, he has chronic anemia, hypertension (HTN), chronic renal insufficiency, and a recently diagnosed 4-cm suprarenal abdominal aortic aneurysm (AAA). Because of his severe CAD, he had to retire from his job as a railroad engineer about 6 months ago. This morning he is being admitted to your telemetry unit for a same-day cardiac catheterization. As you take his health history, you note that his wife died a year ago (about the same time that he had his MI) and that he does not have any children. He is a current cigarette smoker with a 50-pack-year smoking history. As you talk with him, you realize that he has only minimal understanding of the catheterization procedure. His vital signs (VS) are 158/94, 88, 20, and 36.2°C.

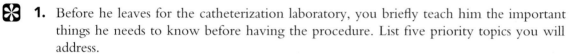 **1.** Before he leaves for the catheterization laboratory, you briefly teach him the important things he needs to know before having the procedure. List five priority topics you will address.

CASE STUDY PROGRESS

Several hours later K.Z. returns from his catheterization. The catheterization report shows 90% occlusion of the proximal left anterior descending (LAD) coronary artery, 90% occlusion of the distal LAD, 70% to 80% occlusion of the distal right coronary artery (RCA), an old apical infarct, and an ejection fraction (EF) of 37%. About an hour after the procedure was finished, you perform a brief physical assessment and find that he now has a grade III/VI systolic ejection murmur at the cardiac apex, crackles bilaterally in the lung bases, and trace pitting edema of his feet and ankles. Except for a soft systolic murmur, these findings were not present before the catheterization.

2. Review the location of the vessels listed in the Case Study Progress on a diagram of the heart from your anatomy book. Sketch (don't trace) a simple illustration of the anterior heart; label the superior and inferior vena cava and the aorta. Draw the main coronary arteries on the surface of the heart. Circle the areas of the LAD and RCA that have significant occlusion. Lightly shade the part of the heart where K.Z. had an earlier infarct. Using the illustration as a patient teaching aid, explain, in plain English, what "37% ejection fraction" means and how you would expect it to influence his everyday activity.

3. What is your evaluation of the catheterization results?

4. What problem do the changes in assessment findings suggest to you? What led you to your conclusion?

✳ **Note:** *Patients usually make statements like, "Something is wrong. . . . I just don't feel right." The nurse needs to be alert to this and reassure the patient that he or she is listening to them and monitoring their status. Such statements should never be taken lightly. They should be shared with nurses on the next shift and the patient's physician. If you have a chance, discuss this with your instructor and the rest of the class.*

5. List four actions you should take as a result of your evaluation of the assessment, and state your rationales.

CASE STUDY PROGRESS

After assessing him, K.Z.'s physician admits him (with a diagnosis of CAD and HF) for coronary artery bypass graft (CABG) surgery. Significant laboratory results drawn at this time are Hct 25.3%, Hgb 8.8 g/dl, BUN 33 mg/dl, and creatinine 3.1 mg/dl. K.Z. is diuresed with furosemide and given 2 units of packed RBCs (PRBCs).

6. Review K.Z.'s health history. Can you identify a probable explanation for his chronic renal insufficiency and anemia?

CASE STUDY PROGRESS

Five days later, after his condition is stabilized, K.Z. is taken to surgery for CABG ×3 V (bypass of 3 coronary arteries). When he arrives in the surgical intensive care unit (SICU), he has a Swan-Ganz catheter in place for hemodynamic monitoring and is intubated. He is put on a ventilator at Fio_2 0.70 and positive end-expiratory pressure (PEEP) at 5 cm H_2O. His first hemodynamic readings are as follows: pulmonary artery pressure (PAP) 41/23 mm Hg, central venous pressure (CVP) 13 mm Hg, pulmonary capillary wedge pressure (PCWP) 13 mm Hg, cardiac index (CI) 1.88 L/min/mm². Arterial blood gases (ABGs) drawn at this time are pH 7.36, Pco_2 46 mm Hg, Po_2 61 mm Hg, and Sao_2 85%, with Hgb 10.3 mg/dl.

7. Why are ABGs necessary in the case of K.Z.? Explain why it would be inappropriate to use pulse oximetry to assess his O_2 saturation status.

8. What is your evaluation of K.Z.'s hemodynamic status based on the previous parameters?

CASE STUDY PROGRESS

Clinically these values show that the pressures within his heart and lungs are a little high and that his CO is a little low. Both these findings indicate that his heart is still having difficulty pumping out all the blood that is returned to it and/or that he is a little fluid overloaded. His condition will require careful monitoring.

9. K.Z. is receiving continuous IV infusions of nitroprusside and dobutamine. He also has just received 2 units of PRBCs. Given this information, do you think the hemodynamic values reported above reflect poor left ventricular function or fluid overload, and why?

10. Why is K.Z. receiving the nitroprusside and dobutamine?

11. What is your responsibility when administering nitroprusside and dobutamine to your patient?

12. Why did he receive 2 units of PRBCs?

13. What is your interpretation of his ABGs on 70% oxygen?

CASE STUDY PROGRESS

After 3 days in the SICU, K.Z.'s condition is stable and he is returned to your telemetry floor. Now, 5 days later, he is ready to go home, and you are preparing him for discharge.

14. List at least two specific areas of teaching that he should receive related to (R/T) his cardiac catheterization.

15. List at least four general areas R/T his CABG surgery in which he should receive instruction before he goes home.

Case Study **14**

Scenario

The wife of C.W., a 70-year-old man, brought him to the emergency department (ED) at 0430 this morning. She told the ED triage nurse that he had had dysentery for the past 3 days and last night he had a lot of "dark red" diarrhea. When he became very dizzy, disoriented, and weak this morning, she decided to bring him to the hospital. C.W.'s vital signs (VS) were 70/– (systolic blood pressure [BP] 70 mm Hg, diastolic BP inaudible), 110, 20. A 16-gauge IV catheter was inserted, and a lactated Ringer's (LR) infusion was started. The triage nurse obtained the following history from the patient and his wife. C.W. has had idiopathic dilated cardiomyopathy (IDCM) for several years. The onset was insidious, but the cardiomyopathy is now severe, as evidenced by an ejection fraction (EF) of 13% found during a recent cardiac catheterization. He experiences frequent problems with heart failure (HF) because of the cardiomyopathy. Two years ago he had a cardiac arrest that was attributed to hypokalemia. He also has a long history of hypertension (HTN) and arthritis. Fifteen years ago he had a peptic ulcer.

An endoscopy showed a 25 × 15 mm duodenal ulcer with adherent clot. The ulcer was cauterized, and C.W. was admitted to the medical intensive care unit (MICU) for treatment of his volume deficit. You are his admitting nurse. As you are making him comfortable, Mrs. W. gives you a paper sack filled with the bottles of medications he has been taking: enalapril (Vasotec) 5 mg PO bid, warfarin (Coumadin) 5 mg/day PO, digoxin 0.125 mg/day PO, KCl 20 mEq PO bid, and tolmetin (an NSAID) 400 mg PO tid. As you connect him to the cardiac monitor, you note that he is in atrial fibrillation (A-fib). Doing a quick assessment, you find a pale man who is sleepy but arousable and oriented. He is still dizzy, hypotensive, and tachycardic. You hear S_3 and S_4 heart sounds and a grade II/VI systolic murmur. Peripheral pulses are all 2+, and trace pedal edema is present. Lungs are clear. Bowel sounds are present, midepigastric tenderness is noted, and the liver margin is 4 cm below the costal margin. A Swan-Ganz catheter and an arterial line are inserted.

1. What medication probably precipitated C.W.'s gastrointestinal (GI) bleeding?

2. What is the most serious potential complication of C.W.'s bleeding?

3. From his history and assessment, identify five signs and symptoms (S/S) (direct or indirect) of GI bleeding and loss of blood volume.

CASE STUDY PROGRESS

C.W. receives a total of 4 units of packed RBCs (PRBCs), 5 units of fresh frozen plasma (FFP), and many liters of crystalloids to keep his mean BP above 60 mm Hg. On the second day in the MICU, his total fluid intake is 8.498 L and output is 3.660 L for a positive fluid balance of 4.838 L. His hemodynamic parameters after fluid resuscitation are pulmonary capillary wedge pressure (PCWP) 30 mm Hg and cardiac output (CO) 4.5 L/min.

4. What is the significance of maintaining a mean BP of 60 mm Hg or greater?

5. Why will you want to monitor his fluid status very carefully?

6. List six things you will monitor to assess C.W.'s fluid balance.

7. Explain the purpose of the FFP for C.W.

CASE STUDY PROGRESS

As soon as you get a chance, you look at C.W.'s admission laboratory results: K 6.2 mmol/L, BUN 90 mg/dl, creatinine 2.1 mg/dl, Hgb 8.4 g/dl, Hct 25%, WBC 16 thou/cmm, and PT 23.4/INR = 4.2. Other results are within the normal range.

8. Are you worried by the elevated potassium (K)? Why, or why not? Explain your answer.

9. In view of the elevated K, what diagnostic test should be performed and why?

10. Why do you think BUN and creatinine are elevated?

11. What do the low hemoglobin (Hgb) and hematocrit (Hct) levels indicate about the rapidity of C.W.'s blood loss?

12. What is the explanation for the prolonged PT/INR?

13. What should be your response to the prolonged PT/INR?

14. What safety precautions should be considered in light of his prolonged PT/INR?

15. How do you account for the elevated WBC count?

CASE STUDY PROGRESS

Mrs. W. has been with her husband since he arrived at the ED and is worried about his condition and his care.

16. List four things you might do to make her more comfortable while her husband is in the MICU.

Case Study **15**

Scenario

J.F. is a 50-year-old married homemaker with a genetic autoimmune deficiency; she has suffered from recurrent bacterial endocarditis. The most recent episodes were a *Staphylococcus aureus* infection of the mitral valve 16 months ago and a *Streptococcus mutans* infection of the aortic valve 1 month ago. During this latter hospitalization, an ECG showed moderate aortic stenosis, moderate aortic insufficiency, chronic valvular vegetations, and moderate left atrial enlargement. Two years ago J.F. received an 18-month course of parenteral nutrition (PN) for malnutrition caused by idiopathic, relentless nausea and vomiting (N/V). She has also had coronary artery disease (CAD) for several years, and 2 years ago suffered an acute anterior wall myocardial infarction (MI). In addition, she has a history of chronic joint pain.

Now, after being home for only a week, J.F. has been readmitted to your floor with endocarditis, N/V, and renal failure. Since yesterday she has been vomiting and retching constantly; she also has had chills, fever, fatigue, joint pain, and headache. As you go through the admission process with her, you note that she wears glasses and has a dental bridge. She is immediately started on PN at 85 ml/hr and on penicillin 2 million units IV piggyback (IVPB) q4h, to be continued for 4 weeks. Other medications are furosemide (Lasix) 80 mg/day PO, amlodipine 5 mg/day PO, potassium chloride (K-Dur) 40 mEq/day PO (dose adjusted according to lab results), metoprolol 25 mg PO bid, and prochlorperazine (Compazine) 2.5 to 5 mg IV push (IVP) prn for N/V. On admission vital signs (VS) are 152/48 (supine) and 100/40 (sitting), 116, 22, 100.2° F. When you assess her, you find a grade II/VI holosystolic (throughout systole) murmur and a grade III/VI diastolic murmur; 2+ pitting tibial edema but no peripheral cyanosis; clear lungs; orientation ×3 but drowsy; soft abdomen with slight left upper quadrant (LUQ) tenderness; hematuria; multiple petechiae on skin of arms, legs, and chest; and splinter hemorrhages under the fingernails.

1. What is the significance of the orthostatic hypotension, the wide pulse pressure, and the tachycardia?

2. What is the significance of the abdominal tenderness, hematuria, joint pain, and petechiae?

3. As you monitor J.F. throughout the day, what other signs and symptoms (S/S) of embolization will you watch for?

4. Three important diagnostic criteria for infectious endocarditis are anemia, fever, and cardiac murmurs. Explain the cause for each sign.

5. On the day after admission, you review J.F.'s laboratory test results: Na 138 mmol/L, K 3.9 mmol/L, Cl 103 mmol/L, BUN 85 mg/dl, creatinine 3.9 mg/dl, glucose 185 mg/dl, WBCs 6.7 thou/cmm, Hct 27%, Hgb 9.0 g/dl. Identify the values that are not within normal ranges, and explain the reason for each abnormality.

6. Which laboratory value(s) reflect(s) catabolism of muscle, and why does muscle catabolism occur?

7. If the PN is scheduled on a 24-hour basis, when would blood glucose be drawn, and why?

8. Why would blood glucose monitoring be important?

9. What is the greatest risk for J.F. during the process of rehydration, and what would you monitor to detect its development?

CASE STUDY PROGRESS

As you admitted J.F., you were aware that as soon as she became stable, she would be going home in a few days on PN and IV antibiotics. The home care agency that will be supervising her care is contacted to coordinate discharge preparations and teaching ASAP.

10. List five important questions in assessing her home health care needs.

CASE STUDY PROGRESS

Fortunately, J.F. has a supportive husband and 2 daughters who live nearby who can function as care-givers when J.F. is discharged. They, along with the patient, will need teaching about endocarditis. Although J.F. has been ill for several years, you discover that she and her family have received little education about the disease. You prepare a teaching plan for the family. The home care agency has a parenteral-enteral nutrition (PEN) team to address her nutritional needs, which will also include vitamins, minerals, and lipids. PN formulations require complex calculations. The PEN team takes care of the formulation of the PN through the pharmacy or dietary staff (depending on local arrangements).

11. List two predisposing causes of bacteremia. Explain.

12. List three other things you would teach.

CASE STUDY PROGRESS
Your hospital discharge planner facilitates J.F.'s transition to home care.

13. During the initial home visit, the home health nurse evaluates J.F.'s IV site for implementation of the IV therapy program. The nurse interviews the family members to determine their willingness to be caregivers and their level of understanding and enlists the patient's and family's assistance to identify 10 teaching goals. What topics would be included on this list?

14. The home health nurse also writes short- and long-term goals for J.F. and her family. Identify two short-term and three long-term goals.

CASE STUDY PROGRESS

Mr. F. and his 2 daughters learned to administer J.F.'s PN during the 18-month treatment. Be aware that IV cases are covered by most insurers on a case-by-case basis and with clear documentation.

15. What documentation would be required to obtain reimbursement? (You need to clearly document everything that is done and why, in detail.)

Case Study **16**

Scenario

You are just getting caught up with your work when you receive the following phone call: "Hi, this is Deb in the emergency department [ED]. We're sending you M.M., a 63-year-old Hispanic woman with a past medical history [PMH] of coronary artery disease [CAD]. Her daughter reports that she's become increasingly weak over the past couple of weeks and has been unable to do her housework. Apparently she has had complaints of [C/O] swelling in her ankles and feet by late afternoon ('she can't wear her shoes') and has nocturnal diuresis ×4. Her daughter brought her in because she has had C/O heaviness in her chest off and on over the past few days but denies any discomfort at this time. The daughter took her to see her family physician, who immediately sent her here. Vital signs [VS] are 146/92, 96, 24, 37.2°C. She has an IV of D_5W at KVO [keep vein open] in her right forearm. Her labs are as follows: Na 134 mmol/L, K 3.5 mmol/L, Cl 103 mmol/L, HCO_3 23 mEq/L, BUN 13 mg/dl, creatinine 1.3 mg/dl, glucose 153 mg/dl, WBC 8.3 thou/cmm, Hct 33.9%, Hgb 11.7 g/dl, platelets 162 thou/cmm. PT/INR, PTT, and urinalysis [UA] are pending. She has had her chest x-ray [CXR] and ECG, and her orders have been written."

1. What additional information do you need from the ED nurse?

2. How are you going to prepare for this patient?

3. Name two types of sphygmomanometers.

4. Monitoring her blood pressure (BP) is going to be important. What would you do to check the cuff and tubing to ensure they are in good working order? List at least three steps.

5. M.M. arrives by wheelchair (W/C). As she transfers from the W/C to the bed, what observations should you make? Why?

6. Given the previous information, which of the following orders can you anticipate as appropriate for this patient? Carefully review each order to determine whether it is appropriate or inappropriate as written. If the order is appropriate, place an "A" in the space provided; if the order is inappropriate, place an "I" in the space provided and change the order to make it appropriate. Also provide any other orders that may be appropriate for this patient.

____ 1. Routine VS
____ 2. Serum magnesium (Mg) STAT
____ 3. Up ad lib
____ 4. 10 g sodium (Na), low–animal fat diet
____ 5. Change IV to normal saline (NS) at 100 ml/hr.
____ 6. Cardiac enzymes on admission and q8h × 24 then daily AM
____ 7. CBC (hemogram), chem 7, and lipid profile in morning
____ 8. Schedule for abdominal CT scan for AM
____ 9. Heparin 10,000 units SC q8h
____ 10. Docusate Na 100 mg/day PO
____ 11. Ampicillin 250 mg IV piggyback (IVPB) q6h
____ 12. Furosemide 200 mg IV push (IVP) STAT
____ 13. Nitroglycerin (NTG) 0.4 mg 1 SL q4h prn for chest pain
____ 14. Schedule echocardiogram

7. When you respond to M.M.'s call light, you observe she is talking rapidly in Spanish and pointing to the bathroom. Her speech pattern indicates she is short of breath (SOB) (she is having trouble completing a sentence without taking a labored breath). You assist her to the bathroom and note that her skin feels clammy. While sitting on the commode, she vomits. On a scale of 0 to 10 (0 being no problem, 10 being a code-level emergency), how would you rate this situation and why?

8. Identify at least four actions you should take next, and state your rationale.

9. The physician calls your unit to find out what is happening. What information would you need to convey at this time?

10. The resident is coming to the floor to evaluate the patient immediately. In the meantime she orders furosemide 40 mg IVP STAT. You have only 20 mg in stock. Should you give the 20 mg now, and then give the additional 20 mg when it comes up from the pharmacy? Explain your answer.

11. M.M. continues to experience vomiting and diaphoresis that are unrelieved by medication and comfort measures. A STAT 12-lead ECG reveals ischemic changes. The patient is transferred to the coronary care unit (CCU). As you give report to the receiving RN, what laboratory value is the most important to report and why?

12. While recovering in the CCU, M.M. slipped in the bathroom and fractured her right humerus. Because of the surgical risks involved, M.M. was treated conservatively and put in a full arm cast. She is placed on prophylactic heparin and is again transferred to your floor. A case manager (CM) has been asked to evaluate M.M.'s home to see whether she can be discharged to her own home or will need to stay in a long-term care facility. Identify at least eight things that the CM would assess.

13. M.M.'s nutritional intake over the past few weeks has been poor. She also has increased nutritional needs because of her fractured arm. What are some of the nutritional needs that should be met? What would you recommend to help her with this?

CASE STUDY PROGRESS

Because the CM determined that M.M. lived in an apartment with poor access, M.M. elects to stay with her daughter and 5 grandchildren in their small home. A home care nurse comes 3 times a week to check on her. M.M. is easily fatigued, and the children are quite lively. School is out for the summer.

14. Suggest some ways the daughter can ensure that her mother isn't overwhelmed and doesn't become exhausted in this situation.

Case Study **17**

Name _____ Class/Group _____ Date _____
Group Members _____

INSTRUCTIONS All questions apply to this case study. Your responses should be brief and to the point. When asked to provide several answers, list them in order of priority or significance. Do not assume information that is not provided. Please print or write clearly. If your response is not legible, it will be marked as ? and you will need to rewrite it.

Scenario

You are in the middle of your shift in the coronary care unit (CCU) of a large urban medical center. Your new admission, C.B., a 47-year-old woman, was just flown to your institution from a small rural community more than 100 miles away. She had an acute anterior wall myocardial infarction (MI) last evening. Her current vital signs (VS) are 100/60, 86, 14. After you make C.B. comfortable, you receive this report from the flight nurse: "C.B. is a full-time homemaker with 4 children. She has had episodes of 'chest tightness' with exertion for the past year, but this is her first known MI. She has a history of hyperlipidemia and has smoked one pack of cigarettes daily for more than 30 years. Surgical history consists of total abdominal hysterectomy (TAH) 10 years ago after the birth of her last child. She has no other known medical problems. Yesterday at 2000 hours she began to have severe substernal chest pain that referred into her neck and down both arms. She rated the pain as 9 or 10 on a 0 to 10 scale. She thought it was severe indigestion and began taking Maalox with no relief. Her husband then took her to the local emergency department [ED], where a 12-lead ECG showed hyperacute ST elevation in the inferior leads II, III, and aV$_F$ and V$_5$ to V$_6$. Before tissue plasminogen activator [TPA] could be given, she went into ventricular fibrillation [V-fib] and was successfully defibrillated after several shocks. She then was given TPA and started on nitroglycerin [NTG], heparin, and lidocaine drips. She also was given IV metoprolol and aspirin 325 mg to chew and swallow. This morning her systolic pressure dropped into the 80s, and she was placed on a dopamine drip and urgently flown to your institution for coronary angiography and possible percutaneous coronary angioplasty [PTCA]. Currently she has lidocaine going at 2 mg/min, heparin at 1200 units/hr, and dopamine at 5 mcg/kg/min. The NTG has been stopped due to low blood pressure [BP]. Lab work done yesterday showed Na 145 mmol/L, K 3.6 mmol/L, HCO$_3$ 19 mmol/L, BUN 9 mg/dl, creatinine 0.8 mg/dl, WBC 14.5 thou/cmm, Hct 44.3%, and Hgb 14.5 g/dl."

1. Given the diagnosis of acute MI, what other lab results are you going to look at?

2. You find the following laboratory results in the patient's chart. For each, interpret the result, and evaluate the meaning for C.B.

   a. Creatinine phosphokinase (CK) levels drawn on admission to the ED and at 4-hour intervals were 95 units/L, 1931 units/L, and 4175 units/L. CK–MB isoenzymes were 5%, 79%, and 216%.

   b. LDL-C: 160 mg/dl

   c. Sao$_2$ on oxygen (O$_2$) at 6 L/min by nasal cannula (NC): greater than 90%.

   d. PT was 11.9 sec/INR = 1.02, both within normal limits (WNL). aPTT before starting heparin was 26.9 sec.

   e. Current magnesium (Mg) level is 2.2 mg/dl; normal level is 1.5 to 3 mg/dl.

   f. Serum potassium (K) was low yesterday (3.6 mmol/L). Current K is 3.9 mmol/L.

3. The 12-lead ECG can tell you the location of the infarction. Look at the leads that show ST elevation (see flight nurse's report). What areas of C.B.'s heart have been damaged?

4. What is tissue plasminogen activator (TPA)? Why is it given, and when is it given to a patient having an MI? How is it administered?

5. An hour after her admission, you are preparing C.B. for her coronary intervention. Evaluate her readiness for teaching and her learning needs. What would you tell her?

CASE STUDY PROGRESS

The following day you care for C.B. again. She is still on the lidocaine and heparin drips. The dopamine has been discontinued. VS are stable. Pulmonary capillary wedge pressure (PCWP) is 20 mm Hg, and cardiac output (CO) is 7.3 L/min. You check her lab results for lidocaine and aPTT levels.

6. The lidocaine level is 2.5 mg/ml, and the aPTT is 40 sec. Analyze the results, and state any actions you would take.

CASE STUDY PROGRESS

As you work with C.B., you notice that she is extremely anxious. You had observed some anxiety yesterday, which you had attributed to the strange CCU environment, pain, and anticipation of the stenting procedure. You know that the stent was successful and that she is physically stable. You wonder what is wrong. She tells you that her MI occurred right in the middle of a move with her family from her rural community to an even smaller and unfamiliar town some 500 miles away in a neighboring state. She is dreading the move. Her husband "becomes angry easily and starts lashing out" toward her and the children. She is afraid to move to a community where she will have no friends and family to support her.

7. How can you help your patient? Evaluate the situation and describe possible interventions.

8. C.B.'s husband comes to visit. He is a handsome, well-dressed man who appears to be loving and attentive toward C.B. He brought a bouquet of roses for her and a box of chocolates for the nurses, "because I appreciate how good you girls have been to my wife." One of your younger colleagues comments to you, "Why, what a nice guy! What is her problem? Every woman would love to be married to a man like that!" How are you going to respond?

chapter
2

Pulmonary Disorders

Case Study 18

Name _____ Class/Group _____ Date _____
Group Members _____

INSTRUCTIONS All questions apply to this case study. Your responses should be brief and to the point. When asked
to provide several answers, list them in order of priority or significance. Do not assume information that is not provided.
Please print or write clearly. If your response is not legible, it will be marked as ? and you will need to rewrite it.

Scenario

You are a public health nurse working at a county immunization and tuberculosis (TB) clinic. B.A. is a
61-year-old woman who wishes to obtain a food handler's license and is required to show proof of a
negative Mantoux (purified protein derivative [PPD]) test before being hired. She came to your clinic
2 days ago to obtain a PPD test for TB. She has returned to have you evaluate her reaction.

1. What is TB, and what microorganism causes it?

* **Hint:** *Information and guidelines about preventing and treating TB can be found on the Centers
for Disease Control and Prevention (CDC) website:* ***http://www.cdc.gov***.

2. What is the route of transmission for TB?

3. The CDC recommends screening people at high risk for TB and providing guidelines for preventive therapy to those at high risk for developing active disease. List five populations at high risk.

4. What is the preferred method for TB screening?

5. What additional information would you want to obtain from B.A. before interpreting her skin test result as positive or negative?

CASE STUDY PROGRESS

B.A. consumes 3 to 4 ounces of alcohol (ETOH) per day and has smoked 1.5 packs of cigarettes per day for 40 years. She is a native-born American, has no risk factors according to the CDC guidelines, lives with her daughter, and becomes angry at the suggestion that she might have TB. She admits that her mother had TB when she was a child but says she has never tested positive. She says, "I feel just fine and I don't think all this is necessary."

6. How do you determine whether the test is positive or negative?

7. You measure and note that the area of erythema measures 30 mm in diameter and the area of induration (hardened tissue) measures 16 mm in diameter. Determine whether B.A.'s skin test is positive or negative.

8. What does a positive PPD result mean?

9. How would you determine whether B.A. has active TB?

CASE STUDY PROGRESS

The physician orders a chest x-ray (CXR) and informs B.A. that her CXR is clear (shows no signs of TB). However, he must report her to the local public health department because her PPD test measured greater than 15 mm. The department will monitor her over time and initiate treatment if she gets TB.

�֍ **10.** According to the CDC, if a person has a positive PPD, what subsequent steps are necessary?

11. According to the American Thoracic Society and CDC (2006) guidelines, what constitutes usual preventive therapy? (NOTE: Be certain to consult the most recent CDC guidelines. Also note that guidelines for diagnosing and treating TB in individuals who are HIV positive are different from those for lower-risk populations.)

12. Different medications are associated with different side effects. Identify the test used to monitor each possible side effect listed below.

    ____ A. Peripheral neuropathy   1. Audiogram

    ____ B. Hepatitis   2. CBC (WBC and platelets)

    ____ C. Fever and bleeding problems   3. Cr/BUN, CrCl (creatinine clearance)

    ____ D. Nephrotoxicity/renal failure   4. Hepatitis C virus (HCV), AST/ALT

    ____ E. Hyperuricemia   5. Physical exam and monofilament testing

    ____ F. Optic neuritis   6. Red-green discrimination and visual acuity

    ____ G. Hearing neuritis   7. Uric acid

13. Nonadherence to drug therapy is a major problem that leads to treatment failure, drug resistance, and continued spread of TB. The CDC recommends 2 methods to ensure compliance with medication for all patients who have drug-resistant TB and those who take medication 2 or 3 times every week. Identify one of those methods.

14. What information should B.A. receive before leaving the clinic?

CASE STUDY PROGRESS
B.A. is hired under the condition that she must immediately report any signs and symptoms (S/S) of active disease to the county health department or her physician and have a yearly CXR.

Case Study **19**

Scenario

M.N., age 40, is admitted with acute cholecystitis, elevated WBC, and a fever of 102° F. She has undergone an open cholecystectomy and has been transferred to your floor. It is the second day postop. She has a nasogastric tube (NGT) to continuous low wall suction, one peripheral IV, and a large abdominal dressing. Her orders are as follows: progress diet to low-fat diet as tolerated; $D_5\frac{1}{2}NS$ with 40 mEq potassium chloride (KCl) at 125 ml/hr; turn, cough, and deep breathe q2h; incentive spirometer (IS) q2h while awake; dangle in AM, ambulate in PM; morphine sulfate 10 mg IM q4h prn for pain; ampicillin (Omnipen) 2 g IV piggyback (IVPB) q6h; chest x-ray (CXR) in AM.

1. Are these orders appropriate for M.N.? State your rationale.

2. What gastrointestinal (GI) complication may result from one of the medications listed in M.N.'s orders?

3. Identify the two most common respiratory-related complications for patients with abdominal or thoracic surgery.

4. What information and assessments would help you differentiate between the two complications in question 3?

5. What procedure is necessary to differentiate between atelectasis and pneumonia?

6. You are assigned to take care of M.N. Her vital signs (VS) are 148/82, 118, 24, 101° F. Her Sao_2 is 88%. Based on these numbers, what do you think is going on with M.N. and why?

7. You know M.N. is at risk for postoperative atelectasis. What is atelectasis, and why is M.N. at risk?

CASE STUDY PROGRESS

After morning report, you do an assessment and auscultate decreased breath sounds and crackles in the right base posteriorly. Her right middle lobe (RML) and right lower lobe (RLL) percuss slightly dull. She splints her right side when attempting to take a deep breath. You suspect that she is developing atelectasis.

8. Identify and clarify five actions you would take next.

9. What four interventions might be used to prevent pulmonary complications?

10. Identify three outcomes that you expect for M.N. as a result of your interventions and her increased activity.

11. M.N.'s sister questions you, saying, "I don't understand. She came in here with a bad gallbladder. What has happened to her lungs?" How would you respond?

12. Radiology calls with a report from the radiologist on the morning CXR. M.N. has atelectasis. Will that change anything that you have already planned for M.N.? Explain what you would do differently if M.N. had pneumonia.

Case Study **20**

Name _____ Class/Group _____ Date _____
Group Members _____
INSTRUCTIONS All questions apply to this case study. Your responses should be brief and to the point. When asked to provide several answers, list them in order of priority or significance. Do not assume information that is not provided. Please print or write clearly. If your response is not legible, it will be marked as ? and you will need to rewrite it.

Scenario

S.R. is a 69-year-old man who owns his own business. The stress of overseeing his employees, meeting deadlines, and carrying out negotiations has led to poor sleep habits. He sleeps 3 to 4 hours a night. He keeps himself going by drinking 2 quarts of coffee and smoking 3 to 4 packs of cigarettes per day. He weighs 280 pounds and does not use alcohol. His wife complains that his snoring has become difficult to live with.

1. As the clinic nurse, what routine information would you want to obtain from S.R.?

CASE STUDY PROGRESS

After interviewing S.R., you report the following information to the provider: blood pressure (BP) 164/90, pulse 92 beats/min, respirations 18 breaths/min, Sao_2 90% on room air. S.R. is under considerable stress, has gained 50 pounds over the past year, and has a history (Hx) of tobacco and caffeine abuse. He complains of (C/O) difficulty staying awake, wakes up with headaches most mornings, and has midmorning somnolence. He is depressed and irritable most of the time and reports difficulty concentrating and learning new things. He has been involved in 3 auto accidents in the past year.

Your examination is normal except for multiple bruises over the right ribcage. You inquire about the bruises, and S.R. reports that his wife jabs him with her elbow several times every night. In her own defense, the wife states, "Well, he stops breathing and I get worried, so I jab him to make him start breathing again. If I don't jab him, I find myself listening for his next breath and I can't go to sleep." You suspect sleep apnea.

2. Identify two of the main types of apnea and explain the pathology of each.

3. Identify at least five signs or symptoms of obstructive sleep apnea (OSA), and star those symptoms that S.R. has.

4. What test(s) help the provider diagnose OSA?

CASE STUDY PROGRESS

The primary care provider (PCP) examined S.R. and documented a long soft palate, recessed mandible, and medium-sized tonsils. S.R.'s overnight screening oximetry study showed 143 episodes of desaturation ranging from 68% to 76%; episodes of apnea were also documented. He was diagnosed with OSA with hypoxemia, and a full sleep study was ordered.

5. The PCP asks you to counsel the patient about lifestyle changes. Name three topics you should address with S.R.

CASE STUDY PROGRESS

S.R. returns for a follow-up (F/U) visit after being diagnosed with OSA. He reports he has lost 10 pounds, but there has been little improvement in his symptoms. He states he fell asleep while driving to work and wrecked his car. He wants to discuss further treatment options.

6. What are the treatment options for OSA? Describe each.

CASE STUDY PROGRESS

S.R. and the PCP decide on the least invasive treatment—continuous positive airway pressure (CPAP). The provider writes a prescription for CPAP. The patient has a choice of which durable medical equipment (DME) company he wants to get his equipment from. You help him by giving him the names of 3 reputable companies and advise him to call his insurance company to find out how much they will pay and how much he will be responsible for.

7. S.R. calls in 2 weeks with C/O dry nasal membranes, nosebleeds, and sores behind his ears. What advice would you give S.R.?

✳ **Note:** *Recipe for Ocean saline spray: Boil water 20 minutes and let cool. Then to 1 quart water add 1 tsp salt plus a pinch of baking soda. Store at room temperature in a covered container for up to 72 hours, then discard.*

✳ **Note:** *Commercial drivers and airline pilots can drive or fly when using CPAP at night, but they must be evaluated for compliance annually.*

Case Study **21**

Scenario

B.T., a 22-year-old man who lives in a small mountain town in Colorado, is highly allergic to dust and pollen; anxiety appears to play a role in exacerbating his asthma attacks. B.T's wife drove him to the clinic when his wheezing was unresponsive to fluticasone (Flovent) and ipratropium bromide (Atrovent) inhalers, he was unable to lie down, and he began to use accessory muscles to breathe. On arrival, his vital signs (VS) are 152/84, 124, 42, 38.0°C. B.T. is started on 4 L oxygen by nasal cannula (O_2/NC), an IV of D_5W at KVO (keep vein open). His arterial blood gases (ABGs) are pH 7.31, $Paco_2$ 48 mm Hg, HCO_3 26 mmol/L, Pao_2 55 mm Hg, Sao_2 88%.

1. Identify the underlying pathophysiology of asthma.

2. The inflammatory response involves what mechanisms?

3. Are B.T.'s VS acceptable? State your rationale.

4. Comment on B.T.'s Sao_2.

5. Identify the drug classifications and actions of fluticasone and ipratropium bromide.

6. Are fluticasone and/or ipratropium appropriate for use during an asthma attack? Explain.

7. The physician orders albuterol 2.5 mg plus ipratropium 250 mcg nebulizer treatment STAT (immediately). What is the rationale for this order?

8. What is the rationale for immediately starting B.T. on O_2?

9. List five short-term interventions that may help relieve B.T.'s symptoms.

CASE STUDY PROGRESS

After several hours of IV and PO rehydration and a second albuterol treatment, B.T.'s wheezing and chest tightness resolve, and he is able to expectorate his secretions. The physician discusses B.T.'s asthma management with him, and the patient says that his inhalers meet his needs on a day-to-day basis but fail him when he has an asthma attack. The physician discharges B.T. with a prescription for oral steroid "burst" (prednisone 40 mg/day ×5 days) and albuterol metered-dose inhaler (MDI) 2 puffs q6h prn using a spacer and recommends that he call the pulmonary clinic for follow-up (F/U) with a pulmonary specialist.

10. What issues would you address in discharge teaching with B.T.?

CASE STUDY PROGRESS

You ask B.T. to demonstrate the use of his MDI. He vigorously shakes the canister, holds the aerosolizer at an angle (pointing toward his cheek) in front of his mouth, and squeezes the canister as he takes a quick, deep breath.

11. What common mistakes has B.T. made when using the inhaler?

12. What would you teach B.T. about the use of his MDI?

✳ **Note:** *Give him written instructions about F/U with the pulmonary specialist.*

13. B.T.'s wife asks about the possibility of B.T. having another attack. How would you respond?

14. If you have a postoperative patient with a history of asthma, what early signs and symptoms (S/S) would indicate respiratory distress? (List at least six.)

15. Identify four S/S of impending respiratory failure.

✳ **Hint:** *To hear lung sounds better, first have the patient turn her or his head to the side (i.e., not facing you) and cough before auscultation.*

✳ **Hint:** *Often asthmatics have little air movement and therefore lungs sound clear. After beta agonist treatment, wheezing may be heard.*

Case Study **22**

Scenario

L.B. is a 30-year-old secretary who is seen with 6 weeks of a dry, hacking cough after recovering from bronchitis this winter. The cough is worse at night and associated with shortness of breath (SOB). In the past she has experienced coughing spells after running a 5K race. She does have hay fever that seems to be year-round and has eczema in the winter. Both of her children and her maternal grand-mother have asthma.

1. As the intake nurse working in the clinic, what routine information would you want to obtain from L.B.?

2. L.B.'s chief complaint (C/C) is a cough. What are the main causes of chronic cough, and what questions should you ask to elicit information about each cause?

CASE STUDY PROGRESS

L.B. denies symptoms in answer to all of your questions except those given in the initial interview. She is not taking any medication other than a multiple vitamin.

3. What would you include in your physical examination and why?

CASE STUDY PROGRESS

L.B. was not in acute distress. Vital signs (VS) were 110/60, 55, 18, peak flow at 350 L/min with good effort ×3. Expected peak flow for her height and age was 512 L/min, so her response is 68% of predicted. She had no sinus tenderness, ears were negative, nasal mucosa was pale and boggy, mouth was negative, there was no cervical adenopathy, lungs were clear to auscultation (CTA), but forced expiration using the peak flow meter (PFM) seemed to generate a cough. Abdomen was soft and nontender. Skin was dry, and hands were erythematous in the web spaces but had no inflammation in the antecubital, trapezius, or popliteal areas (common location of adult eczema).

4. The provider orders a predilator and postdilator pulmonary function test (PFT). What is the purpose of completing the PFTs predilator and postdilator?

5. The diagnosis of asthma is confirmed, and L.B. returns to the clinic for asthma education. What topics should you address?

6. What is a PFM, and what is the purpose of the peak expiratory flow rate (PEFR) measurement?

7. Give L.B. precise instructions to perform the PFM maneuver.

8. The provider ordered triamcinolone (Azmacort) 2 puffs bid and albuterol 2 puffs q6h prn. What points should you include when teaching L.B. about her medications?

9. You instruct L.B. in the proper use of the MDI using a spacer. How would you explain proper MDI use?

CASE STUDY PROGRESS

During a follow-up (F/U) visit, L.B.'s asthma is listed as mild persistent asthma. Her peak flow on the albuterol and triamcinolone has increased to 450 L/min, which is 88% of predicted; her cough has subsided, and she can again participate in sports without problems. There is no nighttime awakening, no loss of work, and no emergency department (ED) visits. She again demonstrates appropriate inhaler technique, has her peak flow record available, and knows that the MDI is empty when the canister floats on its side.

As for triggers, she has noted that wood smoke in the air causes coughing, and she will pretreat with albuterol before exercising outdoors in the winter. Treatment is aimed at avoiding known allergens and respiratory irritants and controlling symptoms and airway inflammation through medication.

Case Study **23**

Scenario

P.R., a 31-year-old woman, contracted an upper respiratory tract infection, developed a high fever, and began to experience progressive ascending paralysis. She was admitted to the local hospital and diagnosed with Guillain-Barré syndrome (GBS). She was intubated and mechanically ventilated. Her vital signs (VS) are 112/68, 134, 12, 101°F. The placement of her percutaneous endoscopic jejunostomy (PEJ) tube was confirmed by abdominal x-ray exam, and she was started on enteral nutrition (EN). The consulting dietitian calculated P.R.'s caloric need at 2800 kcal/24 hr. P.R. is 5'4" and weighs 123 pounds. (NOTE: Registered dietitians [RDs] prefer the "t" spelling rather than "dietician.")

❋**Note:** *A PEJ is a PEG (percutaneous endoscopic gastrostomy) tube with a transjejunal limb.*

1. What is ascending paralysis?

2. Identify and discuss at least two factors that would influence the physician's decision to place P.R. on EN.

3. You note that 2800 kcal/24 hr is a higher than expected caloric requirement for a woman 5'4", 123 pounds. Offer a possible explanation for her current needs.

4. Absolute medical contraindications to enteral feeding are few, and it is preferable to demonstrate failure of EN than to assume that the gastrointestinal (GI) tract is nonfunctional and initiate total parenteral nutrition (TPN). Give three examples of medical diagnoses for which EN would be contraindicated.

5. Pulmonary aspiration is a risk with enteral feedings, although the risk is substantially reduced with jejunum placement. Identify four measures that can be taken to minimize the risk for aspiration.

6. Identify five strategies for preventing bacterial contamination of the feeding formula and tubing.

7. Identify two indicators that an EN infusion rate is too rapid.

8. The nurse needs to monitor P.R.'s GI response to EN and steroid therapy. Identify two observations that need to be recorded, and explain the significance of each.

9. It is a common belief that diarrhea (defined as more than 3 liquid stools per day) is a natural consequence of EN administration. Discuss whether this is a true statement.

10. Identify three factors that could cause diarrhea.

CASE STUDY PROGRESS

As P.R.'s nurse, you are concerned about meeting her needs for fluids, oral hygiene, skin integrity, and activity.

11. Discuss five indicators that would help you assess fluid status.

12. The goal R/T P.R.'s mouth care is to preserve the oral mucosa and dentition. Identify three strategies for providing oral hygiene with an oral endotracheal tube (ETT) in place.

13. What is the rationale for not taking an oral temperature near an ETT?

14. You assess P.R.'s skin every 4 hours. Identify three treatment goals in relation to skin and positioning.

15. What four strategies will facilitate the expected outcome of maintaining skin integrity?

16. You approach P.R. to begin range–of–motion (ROM) exercises. You ask her whether she is experiencing muscle pain at this time, and she nods. You tell P.R. that you will wait until she is pain free to perform the exercises. Why?

CASE STUDY PROGRESS

It takes nearly a year for P.R. to make a full recovery. Note that recovery proceeds from proximal to distal.

Case Study **24**

Scenario

A.B., a 40-year-old man, is admitted to your medical floor with a diagnosis of pleural effusion. He
complains of (C/O) shortness of breath (SOB); pain in his chest; weakness; and a dry, irritating cough.
His vital signs (VS) are 142/82, 118, 38 (labored and shallow), 38.9°C. His chest x-ray (CXR) shows a
large pleural effusion and pulmonary infiltrates in the right lower lobe (RLL) consistent with pneumonitis. (NOTE: When the cause of the lung infection is unknown, the condition should be referred to as
pneumonitis.)

1. Given his diagnosis, are A.B.'s admission VS expected? Explain.

2. What is pleural effusion?

3. What is the difference between transudate and exudate?

4. List three common causes of pleural effusion.

5. Review the pathophysiology and consequences of pleural effusion and pulmonary infiltrates.

6. How does the underlying pathophysiology give rise to A.B.'s presenting signs and symptoms (S/S)?

7. How does A.B.'s increased metabolic rate affect his nutritional needs?

CASE STUDY PROGRESS

The physician performs a thoracentesis and drains 1500 ml of fluid. A specimen for culture and sensitivity (C&S) is sent to the laboratory, and the patient is started on cefuroxime 1 g IV piggyback (IVPB) q8h.

8. What is a thoracentesis?

9. What maneuvers would promote the clearance of pulmonary secretions?

10. The pleural C&S results indicate a large amount of *Klebsiella* organism growth that is sensitive to cefuroxime. What action should you take next?

11. Because fluid continues to collect in the pleural space, the physician decides to insert a pleural chest tube under nonemergent conditions. What is your responsibility as A.B.'s nurse?

12. Evaluate each of the following statements about chest tube drainage systems. Enter "T" for true or "F" for false. Discuss why the false statements are incorrect.

_____ 1. It is the height of the column of water in the suction control mechanism, not the setting of the suction source, that actually limits the amount of suction transmitted to the pleural cavity.

_____ 2. A suction pressure of +20 cm H_2O is commonly recommended for adults.

_____ 3. Bubbling in the water-seal chamber usually means that air is leaking from the lungs, the tubing, or the insertion site.

_____ 4. The rise and fall of the water level with the patient's respirations reflect normal pressure changes in the pleural cavity with respirations.

_____ 5. The chamber is a closed system; therefore water cannot evaporate.

_____ 6 To declot the drainage tubing, put lotion on your hands, compress the tubing, and vigorously strip long segments of the tubing before releasing.

_____ 7. You lower the bed on top of the drainage system and break it. Because you noted an air leak from A.B.'s lung during your initial assessment, you may clamp the chest tube for the short time it takes to reestablish the drainage system.

_____ 8. The chest tube becomes disconnected from the drainage system. Because you noted an air leak from the lung during your initial assessment, you can submerge the chest tube 1 to 2 inches below the surface of a 250 ml bottle of sterile saline or water.

_____ 9. The collection chamber is full, so you need to connect a new drainage system to the chest tube. It is appropriate to momentarily clamp the chest tube while you disconnect the old system and reconnect the new.

_____ 10. The drainage system falls over, spilling the chest drainage into the other drainage columns. The total amount of drainage can be obtained by adding the amount of drainage in each of the columns.

13. How would the nurse appropriately maintain the chest tube system on A.B.?

CASE STUDY PROGRESS

A.B. receives aggressive antibiotic and pulmonary therapy, the chest tube is discontinued (D/C), and he is discharged 3 days later with follow-up (F/U) home care and appointments for F/U clinic visits.

Case Study **25**

Name _____ Class/Group _____ Date _____
Group Members _____

INSTRUCTIONS All questions apply to this case study. Your responses should be brief and to the point. When asked to provide several answers, list them in order of priority or significance. Do not assume information that is not provided. Please print or write clearly. If your response is not legible, it will be marked as ? and you will need to rewrite it.

Scenario

A.W., a 52-year-old woman disabled from severe emphysema, was walking at a mall when she suddenly grabbed her right side and gasped, "Oh, something just popped." A.W. whispered to her walking companion, "I can't get any air." Her companion yelled for someone to call 911 and helped her to the nearest bench. By the time the rescue unit arrived, A.W. was stuporous and in severe respiratory distress. She was intubated, an IV of lactated Ringer's (LR) to KVO (keep vein open) was started, and she was transported to the nearest emergency department (ED).

On arrival at the ED, the physician auscultates muffled heart tones, no breath sounds on the right, and faint sounds on the left. A.W. is stuporous, tachycardic, and cyanotic. The paramedics inform the physician that it was difficult to ventilate A.W. A STAT portable chest x-ray (CXR) and arterial blood gases (ABGs) are obtained. A.W. has an 80% pneumothorax on the right, and her ABGs on 100% oxygen are pH 7.25, $Paco_2$ 92 mm Hg, Pao_2 32 mm Hg, HCO_3 27 mmol/L, base excess (BE) +5 mmol/L, Sao_2 53%.

1. Given the diagnosis of pneumothorax, explain why the paramedic had difficulty ventilating A.W.

2. Interpret A.W.'s ABGs.

3. What is the reason for A.W.'s ABG results?

4. The physician needs to insert a chest tube. What are your responsibilities as the nurse?

5. As the nurse, it is your responsibility to ensure pain control. In A.W.'s case, would you administer pain medication before the chest tube insertion?

6. The ED physician inserts a size 32F chest tube in the sixth intercostal space (ICS), midaxillary line. Would you expect to observe an air leak when A.W.'s chest drainage system is in place and functioning?

7. Would you expect A.W.'s lung to reexpand immediately after the chest tube insertion and initiation of underwater suction? Explain.

8. The clerk tells you A.W.'s husband has just arrived; A.W. will be admitted to the hospital. How would you address this issue with her husband?

9. You approach A.W.'s bedside and ask about what looks like 2 healed chest tube sites on her right chest. A.W.'s husband informs you that this is the third time she has had a collapsed lung. He asks whether this trend will continue. How would you respond?

10. A.W. recovers and is discharged home 4 days later with a chest tube and Heimlich valve. The physician connects a one-way (Heimlich) valve between the distal end of the chest tube and a drainage pouch. Discuss the purpose of this device.

CASE STUDY PROGRESS

A.W. develops several more spontaneous pneumothoraces on the right side and eventually has bleo-mycin instilled over the right lung to induce scarring. She says, "It felt like someone poured kerosene in and threw a lit match in after it. It was the most painful thing I ever went through." Research the scarring procedure so that you know what it does and why it is necessary.

> ✳ **Note:** *Sclerosing a lung doesn't have to feel like it is burning; it should be managed with adequate pain medication.*

Case Study **26**

Name _____ Class/Group _____ Date _____
Group Members _____
INSTRUCTIONS All questions apply to this case study. Your responses should be brief and to the point. When asked to provide several answers, list them in order of priority or significance. Do not assume information that is not provided. Please print or write clearly. If your response is not legible, it will be marked as ? and you will need to rewrite it.

Scenario

The sister of C.K. called to report her 71-year-old brother came down with a fever 2 days ago. Now he has shaking chills, productive cough, and an inability to lie down to sleep because "he can't stop coughing." C.K. is examined at the hospital's primary care clinic, is diagnosed (Dx) with community-acquired pneumonia (CAP), and is admitted to your floor. The intern is busy and asks you to complete your routine admission assessment and call her with your findings.

1. Identify the four most important things to include in your assessment.

CASE STUDY PROGRESS

Your assessment findings are as follows: C.K.'s vital signs (VS) are 154/82, 105, 32, 103°F, Sao$_2$ 84% on room air. You auscultate decreased breath sounds in the left lower lobe (LLL) anteriorly and posteriorly and hear coarse crackles in the left upper lobe (LUL). His nail beds are dusky on fingers and toes. He has cough productive of rust-colored sputum and complains of (C/O) pain in the left side of his chest when he coughs. C.K. seems to be well nourished and adequately hydrated. He is a lifetime nonsmoker and nondrinker. Past medical history (PMH) includes coronary artery disease (CAD) and myocardial infarction (MI) ×2 with a stent ×3; he is currently on metoprolol, amlodipine, lisinopril, and furosemide; for his type 2 diabetes mellitus (DM), he is also taking metformin and rosiglitazone. He reports he has not been sexually active for 15 years but was always monogamous with his wife of 49 years. He has never gotten the Pneumovax or flu shot. He does report getting "hives" when he took "an antibiotic pill" a few years ago but doesn't remember the name of the antibiotic.

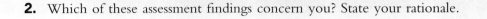

2. Which of these assessment findings concern you? State your rationale.

CASE STUDY PROGRESS

The intern writes the following orders: regular diet; VS with temperature q2h; maintenance IV of D$_5$½NS at 125 ml/hr; ceftriaxone 1 g IV q24h × 10, doxycycline 100 mg bid × 10; titrate oxygen (O$_2$) to maintain oximeter (Sao$_2$) over 90%; obtain sputum for culture and sensitivity (C&S) ×3; draw blood cultures at 2 sites for temperature over 102°F; CBC with differential, basic metabolic panel (BMP), and urinalysis (UA) with C&S as indicated; chest x-ray (CXR) on admission and in the morning.

3. Review the orders and determine what you would do first.

4. Is the IV fluid of D$_5$½NS appropriate for C.K.? State your rationale.

5. What is the rationale for ordering O$_2$ to maintain Sao$_2$ over 90%?

6. What is a C&S test, and why is it important?

7. Why would blood cultures be drawn if the patient spikes a fever?

8. Why are blood cultures drawn from two different sites?

9. What general information can be obtained from a CXR?

10. C.K. recovers from his pneumonia and is preparing for discharge. You know that C.K. is at increased risk for contracting CAP infections. Discuss four strategies for prevention.

11. C.K. confides in you, "You know, my wife died a year ago, and I live alone now. I've been thinking . . . this pneumonia stuff has been a little scary." How will you respond?

✳ **Note:** *Pneumonia, etiology unknown, is properly called pneumonitis. When the term pneumonitis is used, it should be defined according to cause, such as viral pneumonia or Klebsiella pneumoniae.*

Case Study **27**

Name _____ Class/Group _____ Date _____
Group Members _____

INSTRUCTIONS All questions apply to this case study. Your responses should be brief and to the point. When asked to provide several answers, list them in order of priority or significance. Do not assume information that is not provided. Please print or write clearly. If your response is not legible, it will be marked as ? and you will need to rewrite it.

Scenario

P.W., a 33-year-old woman diagnosed with Guillain-Barré syndrome (GBS), is being cared for on a special ventilator unit of an extended care facility because she requires 24-hour-a-day nursing coverage. She has been intubated and mechanically ventilated for 3 weeks and has shown no signs of improvement in respiratory muscle strength. Her ventilator settings are assist-control (A/C) of 12 breaths/min, tidal volume (V_T) 700 ml, Fio_2 0.50, positive end-expiratory pressure (PEEP) 5 cm H_2O. Her vital signs (VS) are 108/64, 118, 12, 38.1°C. She is receiving enteral nutrition by PEJ (percutaneous endoscopic gastrostomy with a transjejunal limb) tube (2800 kcal/24 hr). P.W.'s 3 children, ages 3, 4, and 6, are staying with her sister because her husband has to keep working his full-time job to maintain their medical insurance.

1. Why is P.W.'s ventilator mode on A/C?

2. P.W. is receiving lorazepam (Ativan) 1 mg slow IV push (IVP) q4h to reduce her anxiety. Identify two factors that should be considered when choosing lorazepam for P.W.

3. Identify nine nonpharmacologic strategies that you could use to reduce P.W.'s anxiety, increase her comfort, and reduce the need for lorazepam. Be creative!

4. You give P.W. a bath and note that her cheeks billow outward each time the ventilator delivers a breath. What could cause this phenomenon?

5. You try repositioning P.W., place a stopcock in the inflation valve, auscultate the lungs, check the length of the tube at the lip (the tube had not moved), check the cuff, and note the air pressure is low. You insert more air in the cuff to seal the leak. Over the next 24 hours the leak becomes worse and the ventilator's low exhaled volume alarm repeatedly sounds. What action should you take?

6. The physician elects to insert a no. 8 Shiley tracheostomy tube with a disposable inner cannula. P.W. becomes increasingly anxious after receiving the news. How would you prepare P.W. and her husband for the tracheostomy?

7. P.W. undergoes the tracheostomy procedure without complications. When you return in the morning and assess the new tracheostomy, you note that the trach tape looks tight. You are unable to insert one finger between P.W.'s neck and the trach tape. Discuss whether or not this is problematic.

8. What should your next actions be?

9. You note that the tissue surrounding the incision is edematous. As you palpate the area, your fingers sink into the skin and you auscultate a popping sound through your stethoscope. Is this to be expected?

10. Based on your findings in question 9, what action should you take?

11. That afternoon, a powerful storm causes a power failure. What should you do?

12. You evaluate P.W.'s activity tolerance and note that she desaturates when turned to her right side. You auscultate tubular breath sounds in the entire right lung posteriorly. Based on your knowledge of pathophysiology, explain the probable cause of the desaturation.

CASE STUDY PROGRESS

You notify the physician of the change in P.W.'s breath sounds. The paramedic unit transports P.W. to the hospital, where she is readmitted for recurring pneumonia.

13. P.W.'s husband arrives shortly after the paramedics transport P.W. to the hospital. He collapses into the nearest chair, tears begin to roll down his cheeks, and he says, "It has been almost a month now. Are you sure she will recover?" How would you respond?

CASE STUDY PROGRESS

P.W. undergoes aggressive antibiotic therapy and is discharged to an extended care facility 5 days later. She progresses slowly. It takes nearly 8 months for her to recover, but recovery is complete.

Case Study **28**

Scenario

C.E., a 73-year-old married man and retired railroad engineer, visits his internist complaining: "Whenever I try to do anything, I get so out of breath I can't go on. I think I'm just getting older, but my
wife told me I had to come see you about it." His resting Sao_2 registers 83%. He is sent to the local
hospital for a chest x-ray (CXR) and arterial blood gases (ABGs) to be drawn after resting 20 minutes
on room air. After obtaining the results, the physician calls C.E. and informs him that he has severe
emphysema and must start on continuous oxygen (O_2) therapy.

1. How should C.E.'s chief complaint (C/C) be recorded?

2. What is emphysema?

3. What is the most common cause of emphysema?

4. Based on this information, what questions will you ask about health behaviors?

5. List an authoritative Internet resource of professional and patient or family information on lung disease.

6. Locate and print a patient education handout in the language of your choice and in English on emphysema from one of the Internet sites or a similar resource. Staple it to this assignment.

CASE STUDY PROGRESS

The physician tells C.E. that his office will have a home health equipment company call him to make arrangements to deliver the equipment and educate him in its use. As an RN working for the company, you are assigned to make the initial home visit.

✳ **Note:** *Diagnosis of emphysema is usually made from the CXR, pulmonary function tests, and ABGs on room air. Insurance companies and Medicare usually pay for O_2 only if room air Pao_2 is less than 55 mm Hg. For further information, locate the Centers for Medicare and Medicaid Services (CMS) on the Internet. Look under U.S. Department of Health and Human Services, CMS, for the most recent directives. Look up the Medicare code (number) and information on reimbursement for home treatment of severe emphysema.*

7. How would you prepare for the first visit?

8. What issues would you address with C.E. and his wife?

9. The next time you visit, C.E. complains of (C/O) sores behind his ears. He explains, "That long oxygen tubing seems to take on a life of its own. It twists around and gets caught under doors, chairs, everything. It darn near rips the ears off my head." What can you tell him that could help?

10. You auscultate C.E.'s breath sounds and detect the odor of Vicks VapoRub. When you question C.E. about the use of Vicks, he tells you that he started to apply it in and around his nose to prevent his nose from becoming dry and sore. How would you counsel C.E. and his wife (safety issues)?

CASE STUDY PROGRESS

C.E. elected to use liquid O_2 because it offers more freedom and portability. It is also lighter in weight.

11. Over the next 3 weeks, C.E. seemed to adjust well to his liquid O_2 system. However, one evening he walked to the kitchen for a snack and became increasingly short of breath (SOB). Identify three possible causes.

CASE STUDY PROGRESS

As per your instructions, C.E. removed the nasal cannula (NC), tested the flow against his check, and felt no O_2 flowing from the catheter. He lacked the force and volume required to yell for help and was too SOB to return to the living room to check his O_2 tank. He bent forward with his elbows on the countertop and struggled to breathe. He became more frightened with each passing second, and his breathing became increasingly more difficult. A minute later, C.E.'s wife found him and reconnected his O_2 tubing. C.E. sat at the table for 20 minutes before he could walk back to the living room.

12. Why did C.E. assume the peculiar position at the countertop?

13. A week later you receive a call from C.E.'s wife. She relates the incident from the previous week and tells you that C.E. "doesn't want her out of his sight." She asks you to come to the house and "talk some sense into him." What teaching strategies will you use with C.E. and his wife?

14. C.E.'s wife asks you what her husband can do to help her around the house. She says, "The doctor told him to go home and take it easy. He sits in a chair all day. He won't even get up to get himself a glass of water. I've got a bad hip and this has been very hard on me." How would you address her issue?

15. C.E. states, "You seem to know what you are talking about, so let me ask you something. I wake up with a headache almost every morning. My wife says it's because I snore so loud and don't breathe right when I sleep. Do you know anything about that?" After asking several questions, you inform C.E. that it sounds like he may not be getting enough O_2 at night. Explain the connection between hypoxemia and morning headaches.

CASE STUDY PROGRESS

C.E. seems impressed by your explanation. He asks whether there is anything that can be done for his problem. You inform him that the first step is to identify the problem. You report to the covering health care provider, and an oximetry study is ordered.

You comment that C.E. sounds like he has a cold. He replies, "Oh, our great-grandchildren were over to visit several days ago and they all had snotty noses. I suspect that I'll get it pretty soon. The problem is, every time I get a cold it goes straight to my lungs."

16. What information would you want to review with C.E. and his wife about the signs and symptoms (S/S) of infection and when to seek treatment?

17. What basic hygiene measures can C.E. and his wife take to prevent his developing an infection? (List at least four.)

18. Why is it important for people with lung disease to seek early intervention for infection?

CASE STUDY PROGRESS

C.E. seemed to be managing his emphysema fairly well. His wife had her hip replaced, made a speedy recovery, and was discharged to home. She suddenly died 4 weeks later from a pulmonary embolus. C.E. was panic stricken at her loss. A psychiatric nurse practitioner was requested to work with him.

✳ **Note:** *Stress the importance of a pulmonary rehabilitation program for all patients with moderate to severe lung disease.*

✳ **Note:** *It is important to keep in mind that many home-bound people with chronic illnesses are living a fragile functional independence, depending on the assistance of their partner. When something happens to the partner (death, illness, or stress-related illness), the remaining person is often forced into a nursing home. It is also easier to understand the pressures experienced by the assisting partner: stress-related illnesses, alcoholism, and other forms of substance abuse are not uncommon in these settings, especially when poor community support and inadequate symptom management are factors.*

Case Study **29**

Name _____ **Class/Group** _____ **Date** _____

Group Members _____

INSTRUCTIONS All questions apply to this case study. Your responses should be brief and to the point. When asked
to provide several answers, list them in order of priority or significance. Do not assume information that is not provided.
Please print or write clearly. If your response is not legible, it will be marked as ? and you will need to rewrite it.

Scenario

D.Z., a 65-year-old man, is admitted to a medical floor for exacerbation of his chronic obstructive pulmonary disease (COPD; emphysema). He has a past medical history (PMH) of hypertension (HTN), which
has been well controlled by enalapril (Vasotec) for the past 6 years, and a diagnosis (Dx) of pneumonia
yearly for the past 3 years. He appears as a cachectic man who is experiencing difficulty breathing at
rest. He reports cough productive of thick yellow-green sputum. D.Z. seems irritable and anxious when
he tells you that he has been a 2-pack-a-day smoker for 38 years. He complains of (C/O) sleeping
poorly and lately feels tired most of the time. His vital signs (VS) are 162/84, 124, 36, 102°F, Sao_2
88%. His admitting diagnosis is chronic emphysema with an acute exacerbation, etiology to be
determined.

His admitting orders are as follows: diet as tolerated; out of bed with assistance; oxygen (O_2) to
maintain Sao_2 of 90%; maintenance IV of D_5W at 50 ml/hr; intake and output (I&O); arterial blood gases
(ABGs) in AM; CBC with differential, basic metabolic panel (BMP), and theophylline (Theo-Dur) level on
admission; chest x-ray (CXR) q24h; prednisone 60 mg/day PO; doxycycline 100 mg PO q12h × 10 days,
azithromycin 500 mg IV piggyback (IVPB) q24h ×2 days then 500 mg PO × 7 days; theophylline 300 mg
PO bid; heparin 5000 units SC q12h; albuterol 2.5 mg (0.5 ml) in 3 ml normal saline (NS) and ipratropium 500 mg by nebulizer q4-6h; enalapril 10 mg PO q AM.

1. Explain the pathophysiology of emphysema.

2. Are D.Z.'s VS and Sao_2 appropriate? If not, explain why.

3. Identify three measures you could try to improve oxygenation.

4. Explain the main purpose of the following classes of drugs: antibiotics, bronchodilators, anticholinergics, and corticosteroids.

5. What are two of the most common side effects of bronchodilators?

6. You deliver D.Z.'s dietary tray, and he comments how hungry he is. As you leave the room, he is rapidly consuming the mashed potatoes. When you pick up the tray, you notice that he hasn't touched anything else. When you question him, he states, "I don't understand it. I can be so hungry, but when I start to eat, I have trouble breathing and I have to stop." One theory for the increased work of breathing is based on carbohydrate (CHO) loading. Explain this phenomenon based on your knowledge of the breakdown of CHO.

7. Identify four strategies that might improve his caloric intake.

8. Identify three expected outcomes of D.Z.'s treatment.

9. You notice a box of dark chocolate on D.Z.'s overbed table. He tells you that he wakes at night and eats 4 or 5 pieces of chocolate. Several of your COPD patients have identified a craving for chocolate in the past. What is the basis for this craving?

10. What would you do to address dietary and nutritional teaching needs with D.Z. and his wife?

11. List six educational topics that you need to explore with D.Z.

12. What other health care professional would probably be involved in D.Z.'s treatments and how? What is the licensure or certification status of that profession in the state in which you are practicing?

CASE STUDY PROGRESS

D.Z.'s wife approaches you in the hallway and says, "I don't know what to do. My husband used to be so active before he retired 6 months ago. Since then he's lost 35 pounds. He is afraid to take a bath, and it takes him hours to dress—that's if he gets dressed at all. He has gone downhill so fast that it scares me. He's afraid to do anything for himself. He wants me in the room with him all the time, but if I try to talk with him, he snarls and does things to irritate me. I have to keep working. His medical bills are draining all of our savings, and I have to be able to support myself when he's gone. You know, sometimes I go to work just to get away from the house and his constant demands. He calls me several times a day asking me to come home, but I can't go home. You may not think I'm much of a wife, but quite honestly, I don't want to come home anymore. I just don't know what to do."

13. How would you respond to her statement?

Case Study **30**

Scenario

The ICU nurse calls to give you the following report: "D.S. is a 56-year-old man with a PMH [past medical history] of chronic bronchitis. He quit smoking 12 years ago and exercises regularly. He went to see his physician with complaints of [C/O] increasing exertional dyspnea; a large mass was found in his right lung. Three days ago he underwent an RML [right middle lobe] and RLL [right lower lobe] lobectomy; the pathology report showed adenocarcinoma. He has no neurologic deficits and his vital signs [VS] run 120/70, 110, about 30, and he has been running a fever of 100.2° F. His heart tones are clear, all peripheral pulses are palpable, and he has an IV of $D_5\frac{1}{2}NS$ at 50 ml/hr in his right forearm. He has a right midaxillary chest tube to PleurEvac drain; there's no air leak, and it's draining small amounts of serosanguineous fluid. He has C/O pain at the insertion site, but the site looks good, and the dressing is dry and intact. He's on 5 L oxygen by nasal cannula [O_2/NC]. He refuses pain medication. He's a real nervous guy and hasn't slept since surgery. He'll be there in about 20 minutes."

1. What additional information would you ask the nurse to provide at this time?

CASE STUDY PROGRESS

D.S. is transported by wheelchair (W/C) past the nurses' station to a room at the far end of the hall. You enter his room for the first time to find him sitting on the edge of the bed with his left leg in bed and his right foot on the floor. You introduce yourself and tell him that you are going to be his nurse for the rest of the shift. You note that he keeps rubbing his left hand over the right side of his chest.

2. What issues or problems can you already identify?

3. List four things you would do for D.S.

CASE STUDY PROGRESS
D.S. states, "I have a nephew who rolled his Jeep and busted himself up real bad. He got hooked on those drugs, and I don't want any part of them."

4. How would you respond to D.S.'s statement?

5. Why is D.S. experiencing difficulty using his right arm? Given the type of surgery he underwent, is this expected?

6. You administer morphine sulfate 8 mg IM and tell D.S. that you will return in 30 minutes; 15 minutes later he turns on his call light. When you enter the room, D.S. says, "I think I'm going to throw up." What are the next three things you would do?

7. D.S. states, "I started to feel sick a couple minutes ago. It just kept getting worse until I knew I was going to throw up." Given this information, what do you think is responsible for the sudden onset of nausea?

8. Would it be appropriate to give D.S. a second dose of morphine before reporting his reaction to the physician? State your rationale. Describe your next steps.

9. D.S.'s pain and nausea are under control an hour later. You remove the chest tube dressing and note that the area around the insertion site looks slightly inflamed, the tissue immediately around the tube looks white and moist, and there is scant amount of brown drainage. What action would you take next?

CASE STUDY PROGRESS
The next day, the nurse giving you his report says that D.S. has been driving her crazy all day long. She tells you that he is fine but has been paranoid and demanding. You enter D.S.'s room to see how he is doing and to tell him you are going to be his nurse again today. You note that his head bobs up and his mouth opens, like a fish taking in water, every time he inhales. He says, "I just can't [breath] seem to [breath] get enough [breath] air."

10. Identify six possible problems that D.S. could have that would account for his behavior.

❃ **11.** What actions should you take next? Give your rationale. The instructor should be able to determine whether the rationale is correct. This is a simple issue.

CASE STUDY PROGRESS
D.S.'s respiratory rate is 46 breaths/min; you auscultate slight air movement over the large airways and no breath sounds distal to the third intercostal space (ICS). He's sitting on the side of the bed with his arms hunched up on the overbed table. His gown is in his lap, he is diaphoretic, you note intercostal retractions with inspiration, and all muscles of the upper torso are engaged in respiration.

12. What would you do next?

CASE STUDY PROGRESS

D.S. is successfully resuscitated and transferred to ICU. The physician returns to your floor and compliments you on your clear thinking and fast action. The nurse who gave you his report comes up to you to apologize. She is relatively new and asks you to explain how you know when a patient is in the early and late stages of respiratory difficulty. She states that she wants to learn from her mistakes so that she doesn't put another patient through what D.S. experienced.

13. How would you distinguish between early and late stages of respiratory failure?

Case Study **31**

Name _____ Class/Group _____ Date _____
Group Members _____
INSTRUCTIONS All questions apply to this case study. Your responses should be brief and to the point. When asked to provide several answers, list them in order of priority or significance. Do not assume information that is not provided. Please print or write clearly. If your response is not legible, it will be marked as ? and you will need to rewrite it.

Scenario

G.S., a 36-year-old secretary, was involved in a motor vehicle accident; a car drifted left of center and struck G.S. head-on, pinning her behind the steering wheel. She was intubated immediately after extrication and flown to your trauma center. Her injuries were found to be extensive: bilateral flail chest, torn innominate artery, right hemothorax and pneumothorax, fractured spleen, multiple small liver lacerations, compound fractures of both legs, and probable cardiac contusion. She was taken to the operating room (OR), where she received 36 units of packed RBCs (PRBCs), 20 units of platelets, 20 units of cryoprecipitate, 12 units fresh frozen plasma (FFP), and 18 L of lactated Ringer's (LR) solution. She was admitted to the ICU postop, where she developed adult respiratory distress syndrome (ARDS).

1. What is ARDS?

CASE STUDY PROGRESS

G.S. has been in ICU for 6 weeks, and her ARDS has almost resolved. She is transferred to your unit. You receive the following report: Neurologic: awake, alert, and oriented (AAO) to person and place, she can move both of her arms and wiggle her toes on both feet; cardiovascular (CV): heart tones are clear, vital signs (VS) are 138/90, 88, 26, 37.4°C, bilateral radial pulse 3+, foot pulses by Doppler only; skin: incisions and lacerations have all healed; respiratory: bilateral chest tubes to water suction with closed drainage, dressings are dry and intact; gastrointestinal (GI): duodenal feeding tube in place; genitourinary (GU): Foley catheter to down drain.

2. What additional information should you require during this report?

CASE STUDY PROGRESS

You complete your assessment of G.S. You note shortness of breath (SOB), crackles throughout all lung fields posteriorly and in both lower lobes anteriorly, and rhonchi over the large airways.

3. What is the significance of crackles and rhonchi in G.S.'s case?

4. The nurse from the previous shift charted the following statement: "Crackles and rhonchi clear with vigorous coughing." Based on your knowledge of pathophysiology, determine the accuracy of this statement.

5. It is time to administer furosemide (Lasix) 40 mg IV push (IVP). What effect, if any, will furosemide have on G.S.'s breath sounds?

6. What action should you take before giving the furosemide?

CASE STUDY PROGRESS

The 0500 laboratory values are as follows: Na 129 mmol/L; K 3.3 mmol/L; Cl 92 mmol/L; HCO_3 26 mmol/L; BUN 37 mg/dl; creatinine 2 mg/dl; glucose 128 mg/dl; Ca 7.1 mg/dl; arterial blood gases (ABGs) on 6 L O_2 by nasal cannula (NC): pH 7.38, $Paco_2$ 49 mm Hg, Pao_2 82 mm Hg, HCO_3 36 mmol/L, BE (base excess) +2.2, Sao_2 91%.

7. Keeping in mind that you are about to administer furosemide, which laboratory values concern you and why?

8. Given the laboratory values listed, what action would you take before administering the furosemide, and why?

CASE STUDY PROGRESS

The physician prescribes the following: draw STAT magnesium (Mg) level; if below 1.4 mg/dl, give magnesium sulfate 3 g in 100 ml normal saline (NS) over 3 hours; give KCl 40 mEq in 100 ml NS IV piggyback (IVPB) over 4 hours now; and give calcium gluconate 2 g in 100 ml NS IVPB over 3 hours. The laboratory is called to draw a STAT Mg level.

9. Given that potassium chloride (KCl) and calcium gluconate are compatible, would you mix them in the same bag of NS? State your rationale.

10. You open G.S.'s medication drawer to draw the furosemide into a syringe. You find one 20-mg ampule. The pharmacist tells you that it will be at least an hour before he can send the drug to you. You realize it is illegal to take medication dispensed by a pharmacist for one patient and use it for another patient. What should you do?

� 11. While you administer the furosemide and hang the IVPB medication, G.S. says, "This is so weird. A couple times this morning, I felt like my heart flipped upside down in my chest, but now I feel like there's a bird flopping around in there." What are the first two actions you should take next? Give your rationale.

12. G.S.'s pulse is 66 beats/min and irregular. Her blood pressure (BP) is 92/70 mm Hg, and respirations are 26 breaths/min. She admits to being "a little lightheaded" but denies having pain or nausea. Your co-worker connects G.S. to the code cart monitor for a "quick look." You are able to distinguish normal P–QRS–T complexes, but you also note approximately 22 very wide complexes per minute. The wide complexes come early and are not preceded by a P wave. What do you think has happened to G.S.?

✖ 13. What should your next actions be?

14. What are the most likely causes of the abnormal beats?

15. You notice that G.S. looks frightened and is lying stiff as a board. How would you respond to this situation?

CASE STUDY PROGRESS

G.S.'s PVCs responded well to treatment. Unfortunately, 1 week later she threw a large embolus. All attempts at resuscitation failed.

chapter 3

Musculoskeletal Disorders

Case Study 32

Name _____ Class/Group _____ Date _____
Group Members _____
INSTRUCTIONS All questions apply to this case study. Your responses should be brief and to the point. When asked
to provide several answers, list them in order of priority or significance. Do not assume information that is not provided.
Please print or write clearly. If your response is not legible, it will be marked as ? and you will need to rewrite it.

Scenario

M.S., a 72-year-old white woman, comes to your clinic for a complete physical examination. She has
not been to a provider for 11 years because "I don't like doctors." Her only complaint today is "pain
in my upper back." She describes the pain as sharp and knifelike. The pain began approximately 3
weeks ago when she was getting out of bed in the morning and hasn't changed at all. M.S. rates her
pain as 6 on a 0- to 10-point pain scale and says the pain decreases to 3 or 4 after taking "a couple
of ibuprofen." She denies recent falls or trauma.

M.S. admits she needs to quit smoking, lose some weight, and start exercising but states, "I don't
have the energy to exercise." She has smoked 1 to 2 packs of cigarettes per day since she was 17
years old. Her last blood work was 11 years ago, and she can't remember the results. She went through
menopause at the age of 47 and has never taken hormone replacement therapy.

The physical exam was unremarkable other than moderate tenderness to deep palpation over the
spinous process at T7. No masses or tenderness to the tissue surrounded the tender spot. No visible
masses, skin changes, or erythema were noted. Her neurologic exam is intact, and no muscle wasting
is noted.

1. An x-ray examination of the thoracic spine reveals osteopenic changes at T7. What does
   this mean?

2. The physician suspects osteoporosis. List seven risk factors associated with osteoporosis.

3. Place a star next to those risk factors specific to M.S.

CASE STUDY PROGRESS

M.S. has never had osteoporosis screening. She confides that her mother and grandmother were diagnosed with osteoporosis when they were in their early 50s.

4. What tests could be done to determine whether M.S. has osteoporosis? Which test is recommended and why?

5. M.S.'s DEXA scan revealed a bone density of −2.6 SD (standard deviations). What does this mean?

6. The physician orders alendronate (Fosamax) 70 mg/wk. What instructions should you give M.S. regarding alendronate?

7. What nonpharmacologic interventions should you teach M.S. to prevent further bone loss?

✳ **Note:** *Many cases of osteoporosis in older women and men develop secondary to gastric problems, renal disorders, arthritis, and medication intake. Also, deficit in calcium intake is relatively common among low-income people with poor nutrition or in elderly individuals living alone.*

CASE STUDY PROGRESS
M.S. seems overwhelmed and says, "I cannot possibly stop smoking and lose weight and exercise all at the same time."

8. You encourage M.S. to start working on one problem at a time. Which problem should M.S. attempt first?

For more information contact:

National Library of Medicine: *http://www.nlm.nih.gov*

NIH Osteoporosis and Related Bone Diseases National Resource Center (ORBD-NRC): *http://www. niams.nih.gov/Health_Info/Bone;* (800) 624-2663

Case Study **33**

Scenario

J.C. is a 41-year-old man who comes to the emergency department (ED) with complaints of (C/O) acute low back pain. He states that he did some heavy lifting yesterday, went to bed with a mild backache, and awoke this morning with terrible back pain. He admits to having had a similar episode of back pain "after I lifted something heavy at work." J.C. has a past medical history (PMH) of peptic ulcer disease (PUD) related to (R/T) NSAIDs use. He is 6′ tall, weighs 265 pounds, and has a prominent "potbelly."

1. J.C. used to take piroxicam (Feldene) 20 mg until he developed his duodenal ulcer. What is the relationship between the two? What signs and symptoms (S/S) would you expect if an ulcer developed?

2. What observable characteristic does J.C. have that makes him highly susceptible to low back injury?

3. What questions would be appropriate to ask J.C. in evaluating the extent of his back pain and injury?

CASE STUDY PROGRESS

All serious medical conditions are ruled out, and J.C. is diagnosed with lumbar strain. The midlevel provider orders a physical therapy (PT) consult to develop a home stretching and back-strengthening exercise program and a dietary consult for weight reduction. J.C. is given prescriptions for cyclobenzaprine (Flexeril) 10 mg tid prn ×3 days only, and celecoxib (Celebrex) 100 mg/day for 3 months. He receives the following instructions: ice packs to the lower back for 20 minutes every hour, no twisting or unnecessary bending, and no lifting more than 10 pounds. J.C. is instructed to rest his back for 1 or 2 days, getting up only now and then to move around to relieve muscle spasms in his back and strengthen his back muscles. He is given an excuse to stay off work for 5 days only, and he is instructed to return to the emergency department (ED) if he gets worse.

4. Why do you think that cyclobenzaprine was prescribed instead of carisoprodol or diazepam?

5. What points would you include when teaching J.C. about muscle relaxants?

6. A PT teaches J.C. maintenance exercises he can do on his own to promote back health. Identify two common exercises that would be included.

7. What is celecoxib, and how does it work? What advantage does this medication have over the "older" NSAIDs?

8. Why would J.C. want to use an NSAID rather than acetaminophen for pain?

For more information contact:

Mayo Clinic: *http://www.mayoclinic.com*

National Institute of Neurological Disorders and Stroke: *http://www.ninds.nih.gov/disorders/ backpain/backpain.htm*

Case Study **34**

Scenario

D.M., a 25-year-old man, hops into the emergency department (ED) with complaints of (C/O) right ankle pain. He states that he was playing basketball and stepped on another player's foot, inverting his ankle. You note swelling over the lateral malleolus down to the area of the fourth and fifth metatarsals, and pedal pulses are 3+ bilaterally. His vital signs (VS) are 124/76, 82, 18. He has no allergies and takes no medication. He states he has had no prior surgeries or medical problems.

1. When assessing D.M.'s injured ankle, what should be evaluated?

2. What should initial management of the ankle involve to prevent further swelling and injury?

3. You note significant swelling over the fourth and fifth metatarsals. How would you further evaluate this finding?

CASE STUDY PROGRESS

X-ray results are negative for fracture, and a third-degree sprain is diagnosed. The physician orders an ankle splint with elastic wrap and crutches with instructions. The physician instructs D.M. not to bear weight on his ankle for 2 days.

4. Describe the technique for applying an elastic wrap. Give the rationale.

5. When instructing D.M. to use crutches, which part of his body should you tell him to rest his weight on while the crutch is bearing the weight? Explain why.

6. You are to instruct D.M. on application of cold and heat, activity, and care of the ankle. What would be appropriate instructions in these areas?

7. D.M. is given a prescription for acetaminophen-hydrocodone (Lortab) for pain. What instructions concerning this medication should you give him on discharge?

8. Four days later D.M. hobbles into the ED and boldly informs you that he "did it again, only this time it was touch football." He states that the pain pills worked so well, he thought it would be OK. You detect the odor of beer on his breath. What are you going to do?

9. You remove his sock and find a large hematoma forming on the lateral aspect of an already swollen ankle. The ankle also shows the color of a bruise that is several days old. You inquire about D.M.'s pain perception. He states, "It doesn't feel too bad now, but I sure saw stars when it popped." What is the significance of his statement?

Case Study **35**

Name _____ Class/Group _____ Date _____
Group Members _____

INSTRUCTIONS All questions apply to this case study. Your responses should be brief and to the point. When asked to provide several answers, list them in order of priority or significance. Do not assume information that is not provided. Please print or write clearly. If your response is not legible, it will be marked as ? and you will need to rewrite it.

Scenario

S.P. is admitted to the orthopedic ward. She has fallen at home and has sustained an intracapsular fracture of the hip at the femoral neck. The following history is obtained from her: she is a 75-year-old widow with 3 children living nearby. Her father died of cancer at 62 years of age (yoa); mother died of heart failure (HF) at 79 yoa. Her height is 5'3", weight 118 pounds. She has a 50-pack-year smoking history and denies alcohol use. She has severe rheumatoid arthritis (RA), had an upper gastrointestinal (UGI) bleed in 1993, and had coronary artery disease (CAD) with coronary artery bypass graft (CABG) 9 months ago. Since that time she has engaged in "very mild exercises at home." Vital signs (VS) are 128/60, 98, 14, 37.2°C, Sao$_2$ 94% on 2 L oxygen by nasal cannula (O$_2$/NC). Her medications are rabeprazole (Aciphex) 20 mg/day, prednisone (Deltasone) 5 mg/day PO, and methotrexate (Amethopterin) 2.5 mg/wk.

1. List four risk factors for hip fractures.

2. Place a star next to each of the responses in question 1 that represent S.P.'s risk factors.

CASE STUDY PROGRESS

S.P. is taken to surgery for a total hip replacement. Because of the intracapsular location of the fracture, the surgeon chooses to perform an arthroplasty rather than internal fixation. The postoperative orders include:

- Cefazolin (Kefzol) 1000 mg IV q8h × 3 doses
- Enoxaparin (Lovenox) 30 mg SC q12h
- Warfarin (Coumadin) 1 to 10 mg/day PO per sliding scale (may or may not be held day of surgery)
- Docusate and senna (Peri-Colace) 1 capsule PO bid
- Multivitamin with iron (Trinsicon) 1 capsule/day PO with meals
- CBC in morning after blood reinfusion
- Hydromorphone (Dilaudid) 25 mg IV by patient-controlled analgesia (PCA) pump
- Physical therapy (PT) and occupational therapy (OT) to evaluate on postoperative day (POD) 1 and start therapy
- Ketorolac (Toradol) 15 mg IM or IV q6h prn ×5 days only
- Hip precautions per protocol
- Ondansetron 4 mg IV q6h prn for nausea
- Toilet seat extension
- Straight catheterization if the patient has not voided by 8 hours postoperatively

3. Why is the patient receiving enoxaparin and warfarin?

4. What is the difference between arthroplasty and open reduction and internal fixation (ORIF)?

5. List four critical potential postoperative problems for S.P.

6. How would you monitor for excessive postoperative blood loss?

7. How should a nurse manage a patient using a blood reinfusion system?

8. According to the lateral traditional surgical approach, there are two main goals for maintaining proper alignment of S.P.'s operative leg. What are they, and how are they achieved?

9. Postoperative wound infection is a concern for S.P. Describe what you would do to monitor S.P. for wound infection.

10. Taking S.P.'s RA into consideration, what interventions should be implemented to prevent complications secondary to immobility?

11. What predisposing factor, identified in S.P.'s medical history, places her at risk for infection, bleeding, and anemia?

12. Briefly discuss S.P.'s nutritional needs.

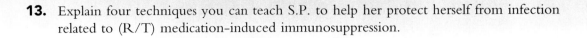

13. Explain four techniques you can teach S.P. to help her protect herself from infection related to (R/T) medication–induced immunosuppression.

CASE STUDY PROGRESS

Discharge planning should begin when the patient is admitted. The case manager (CM) or social worker will work with the family to initiate placement in a rehabilitation facility.

14. What factors need to be taken into consideration when choosing a rehabilitation facility?

CASE STUDY PROGRESS

S.P. is admitted to the rehabilitation facility close to one daughter's home; she completed rehab and is discharged to home. Her daughter still looks in on her every day.

Case Study **36**

Scenario

H.K. is a 26-year-old man who tried to light a cigarette while driving and lost control of his Jeep. The Jeep flipped and landed on the passenger side. H.K. was transported to the emergency department (ED) with a deformed, edematous right lower leg and a deep puncture wound approximately 5 cm long over the deformity. Blood continues to ooze from the wound.

1. What further assessment should the nurse make of the leg injury, and what precautions should he or she take in making this assessment?

2. What would be the most appropriate method for controlling bleeding at this wound site?

3. From the above information, it is clear that H.K. is a smoker. List at least three issues related to (R/T) his smoking that can complicate his care and recovery. What interventions could be instituted to counter these complications? Would using a nicotine patch eliminate these problems?

4. What is the best way to immobilize the leg injury before surgery?

CASE STUDY PROGRESS

H.K. is taken to surgery for open reduction and internal fixation (ORIF) of the tibia and fibula fractures. He returns with a full-leg fiberglass cast with windows over the areas of surgery.

5. Describe assessment of a patient with a long leg cast involving trauma and surgery.

6. In assessing H.K.'s cast on the third day postop, you notice a strong foul odor. Drainage on the cast is extending, and H.K. is complaining of (C/O) pain more often and seems considerably more uncomfortable. Vital signs (VS) are 123/78, 102, 18, 102.2° F. What is your analysis of these findings?

CASE STUDY PROGRESS

H.K. returns to surgery. The wound over H.K.'s fracture site has become necrotic with purulent drainage. The wound is debrided and cultured; then a posterior splint is applied. H.K. returns to his room with orders for wet-to-moist dressing changes. The physician suspects osteomyelitis and orders nafcillin (Unipen) and ciprofloxacin (Cipro).

7. As you continue to assess H.K. over the following days, what evidence will you look for that antibiotics are effectively treating the infection?

8. What should H.K. be taught concerning the care of his cast?

9. What nutritional needs will H.K. have, and why?

10. To ensure pain management, H.K. is given a fentanyl TTS 75 mcg/hr transdermal patch. What therapeutic category does this drug belong to? What signs and symptoms (S/S) would you see if he were to have a toxic or overdose reaction?

11. What is the antidote to toxic narcotic reactions, and how is it administered?

12. What issues would the discharge planner need to address with H.K.?

CASE STUDY PROGRESS

H.K. stayed in his apartment with a loan from his parents. Friends drove him to physical therapy (PT) on their way to class at the university and took him back on their way home. He managed well and went back to work while still in his cast.

Case Study **37**

Name _____ Class/Group _____ Date _____
Group Members _____

INSTRUCTIONS All questions apply to this case study. Your responses should be brief and to the point. When asked to provide several answers, list them in order of priority or significance. Do not assume information that is not provided. Please print or write clearly. If your response is not legible, it will be marked as ? and you will need to rewrite it.

Scenario

M.M., a 76-year-old retired schoolteacher, underwent open reduction and internal fixation (ORIF) for a fracture of his right femur. His preoperative control prothrombin time (PT) was 11 sec. He has been on bed rest for the first 2 days postoperatively. At 0600 his vital signs (VS) were 132/84, 80 with regular rhythm, 18 unlabored, and 37.2° C. He is awake, alert, and oriented (AAO) with no adventitious heart sounds. Breath sounds are clear but diminished in the bases bilaterally. Bowel sounds are present, and he is taking sips of clear liquids. An IV of $D_5\frac{1}{2}NS$ is infusing TKO (to keep open) in his left hand and should be saline locked in the AM if he is able to maintain adequate PO fluid intake. He has orders for oxygen (O_2) to maintain Sao_2 over 90%. His lab work shows Hct 34%, Hgb 11.3 mg/dl, K 4.1 mmol/L, PTT 44 sec. Pain is controlled with morphine sulfate 4 mg IV and promethazine (Phenergan) 25 mg IV q3h. He is also taking heparin 5000 units SC bid, taking docusate sodium, and wearing a nitroglycerin patch.

At 2330 on the second postoperative day, you answer M.M.'s call light and find him lying in bed breathing rapidly and rubbing the right side of his chest. He is complaining of (C/O) right-sided chest pain and appears to be restless.

1. What are you going to do?

CASE STUDY PROGRESS

He is slightly hypotensive, tachycardic, tachypneic, restless, and slightly confused. The pulse oximeter reads 86%, so you start him on 3 to 6 L O_2 by nasal cannula (NC). You identify faint crackles in the posterior bases bilaterally; they were clear this morning. The monitor shows nonspecific T wave changes and tachycardia.

2. Based on your findings, you call the physician. What information are you going to give him or her?

3. The physician orders that the patient be transferred to ICU and have blood coagulation studies, arterial blood gases (ABGs) on room air, continuous pulse oximetry, STAT chest x-ray (CXR), and STAT 12-lead ECG. What information will the physician gain from each of the above?

4. Why would the physician order ABGs on room air as opposed to with supplemental O_2?

CASE STUDY PROGRESS

The ABGs return as follows: pH 7.55, $Paco_2$ 24 mm Hg, HCO_3 24 mmol/L, and Pao_2 56 mm Hg at sea level. Sao_2 is 86% on room air. CXR shows a small right infiltrate. VS are 150/92, 110, 28, 37.2°C.

5. What is your interpretation of the ABGs, and what do you think the physician will order next?

6. The V/Q is performed, and the interpretation reads "strongly suggestive of a PE." What are the most likely sources of the embolus?

7. Before the latest PTT/INR results are back, the physician orders a heparin bolus of 5000 units IV followed by an infusion of 1200 units/hr. The lab calls with a critical value—the PTT is 120 sec. Based on these results, what action would you take?

CASE STUDY PROGRESS
The PTT 4 hours later is 29 sec.

8. The next day the physician's orders read, "Coumadin 2.5 mg, PT/INR in AM; DC [discontinue] heparin." What is wrong with these orders?

9. Thrombolytics, such as alteplase and urokinase, have been beneficial in the treatment of PE. Why would these medications be contraindicated in M.M.'s case?

10. List three priority problems related to (R/T) the care of M.M. in his current situation.

11. Several days later you hear M.M. asking his son to bring in a "decent razor" because he is tired of the stubble left by the unit's shaver. How would you address this issue?

Case Study **38**

Scenario

J.F., a 67-year-old woman, was involved in an auto accident and is life-flighted to your facility. She sustained a ruptured spleen, fractured pelvis, and compound fractures of the left femur. On admission (5 days ago) she underwent a splenectomy. Her pelvis was stabilized with an external fixation device 3 days ago, and yesterday her left femur was stabilized using balanced suspension with skeletal traction. She has a Thomas ring with Pearson attachment on her left leg. She has 20 pounds of skeletal traction and 5 pounds applied to the balanced suspension. Her left femur is elevated off the bed at approximately 45 degrees. The foreleg (lower part of her leg) is parallel to the bed and lies in a sling that the nurse adjusts on the frame, and the foot hangs freely. This morning J.F. was transferred to your orthopedic unit for specialized care. You are the nurse assigned to care for her on the night shift.

1. You enter J.F.'s room for the first time. What aspects of the traction would you want to inspect?

2. When inspecting the skeletal pin sites, you note that the skin is reddened for an inch around the pin on both the medial and lateral left leg. What does this finding indicate, and what action would you take?

3. You find J.F.'s body in the lower 75% of the bed, her left upper leg at an exaggerated angle (more than 45 degrees). The knot at the end of the bed is caught in the pulley, and the 20-pound weight is dangling just above the floor. What are you going to do?

4. When you lift J.F., you notice that her sheets are wet. Because you have lots of help in the room, you decide to change J.F.'s linen. How would you accomplish this task?

5. J.F. tells you that she feels like she needs to have a bowel movement (BM), but it is too painful to sit on the bedpan. How would you respond?

6. J.F. expels a few small, hard, round pieces of stool. What could be done to promote normal elimination?

CASE STUDY PROGRESS
You ask J.F. if she is ready for her bath, and she responds positively. You let her bathe the parts she can reach and engage her in a conversation as you attend to the rest of her body. While performing perineal care, you notice that the folds of skin around her perineal area are reddened and excoriated.

7. Given that J.F. has been on antibiotics for the past 5 days, what is the likely cause of the problem, and what needs to be done to encourage healing?

8. You ask J.F. what she is doing to exercise while she is confined to bed. She looks surprised and states that she isn't doing anything. What activities can J.F. engage in while on bed rest?

9. You realize that maintaining skin integrity is a challenge in J.F.'s case. What measures will you take to prevent skin breakdown?

10. Although J.F. is recovering nicely, she is becoming increasingly withdrawn. You enter her room and find her crying. She tells you that she is all alone here, that she misses her family terribly. You know that her son is flying into town tomorrow but will only be able to stay a few days. What can be done so that J.F. benefits from her family support system?

Case Study **39**

Name _____ **Class/Group** _____ **Date** _____
Group Members _____

INSTRUCTIONS All questions apply to this case study. Your responses should be brief and to the point. When asked to provide several answers, list them in order of priority or significance. Do not assume information that is not provided. Please print or write clearly. If your response is not legible, it will be marked as ? and you will need to rewrite it.

Scenario

You are working in the emergency department (ED) when M.C., an 82-year-old widow, arrives by ambulance. Because M.C. had not answered her phone since noon yesterday, her daughter went to her home to check on her. She found M.C. lying on the kitchen floor, incontinent of urine and stool, with complaints of (C/O) pain in her right hip. Her daughter reports a past medical history (PMH) of hypertension (HTN), angina, and osteoporosis. M.C. takes propranolol (Inderal), nitroglycerin patch, indapamide (Lozol), and conjugated estrogen (Premarin) daily. The daughter reports that her mother is normally very alert and lives independently. On examination you see an elderly woman, approximately 100 pounds, holding her right thigh. You note shortening of the right leg with external rotation and a large amount of swelling at the proximal thigh and right hip. M.C. is oriented to person only and is confused about place and time. M.C.'s vital signs (VS) are 90/65, 120, 24, 97.5° F; her Sao_2 is 89%. She is profoundly dehydrated. Preliminary diagnosis is fracture of the right hip.

1. In view of M.C.'s history of HTN and the fact that she has been without her medications for at least 24 hours, explain her current VS.

�֍ **2.** Based on her history and your initial assessment, what three priority interventions should be initiated?

3. M.C.'s daughter states, "Mother is always so clear and alert. I have never seen her act so confused. What's wrong with her?" What are three possible causes for M.C.'s disorientation that should be considered and evaluated?

CASE STUDY PROGRESS

X-ray films confirm the diagnosis of intertrochanteric femoral fracture. Knowing that M.C. is going to be admitted, you draw admission labs and call for the orthopedic consult.

4. What laboratory and diagnostic studies would be ordered to evaluate M.C.'s condition, and what critical information will each give you?

5. What are the five P's that should guide the assessment of M.C.'s right leg before and after surgery?

6. In evaluating M.C.'s pulses, you find her posterior tibial pulse and dorsalis pedis pulse to be weaker on her right foot than on her left. What could be a possible cause of this finding?

7. In planning further care for M.C., list four potential complications for which M.C. should be monitored.

8. M.C. keeps asking about "Peaches." No one seems to be paying attention. You ask her what she means. She says Peaches is her little dog, and she's worried about who is taking care of it. How will you answer?

CASE STUDY PROGRESS
M.C. is placed in Buck's traction and sent to the orthopedic unit until an open reduction and internal fixation (ORIF) can be scheduled. Hydrocodone-acetaminophen (Lortab) is ordered for severe pain with orders for acetaminophen and tramadol for mild and moderate pain, respectively. M.C.'s cardiovascular, pulmonary, and renal status is closely monitored.

9. Tramadol and Lortab are both constipating. What would you do to prevent constipation?

10. What is obstipation?

CASE STUDY PROGRESS

After her surgery, M.C. is transferred to a long-term care facility for physical and occupational therapy rehabilitation. She is placed on prophylactic warfarin (Coumadin).

Case Study **40**

Scenario

E.B., a 69-year-old man with type 1 diabetes mellitus (DM), is admitted to a large regional medical center complaining of (C/O) severe pain in his right foot and lower leg. The foot and lower leg are cool and without pulses (absent by Doppler). Arteriogram demonstrates severe atherosclerosis of the right popliteal artery with complete obstruction of blood flow. Despite attempts at endarterectomy and administration of intravascular alteplase (tissue plasminogen activator [TPA]) over several days, the foot and lower leg become necrotic. Finally, the decision is made to perform an above-the-knee amputation (AKA) on E.B.'s right leg. E.B. is recently widowed and has a son and daughter who live nearby. In preparation for E.B.'s surgery, the surgeons wish to spare as much viable tissue as possible. Hence an order is written for E.B. to undergo 5 days of hyperbaric therapy for 20 minutes bid.

1. What is the purpose of hyperbaric therapy?

CASE STUDY PROGRESS

As you prepare E.B. for surgery, he is quiet and withdrawn. He follows instructions quietly and slowly without asking questions. His son and daughter are at his bedside, and they also are very quiet. Finally, E.B. tells his family, "I don't want to go like your mother did. She lingered on and had so much pain. I don't want them to bring me back."

2. You look at his chart and find no advance directives. What is your responsibility?

3. What is your assessment of E.B.'s behavior at this time?

4. What are some appropriate interventions and responses to E.B.'s anticipatory grief?

CASE STUDY PROGRESS

E.B. returns from surgery with the right stump dressed with gauze and an elastic wrap. The dressing is dry and intact, without drainage. He is drowsy with the following vital signs (VS): 142/80, 96, 14, 97.9°F, Sao₂ 92%. He has a maintenance IV of D₅.9NS infusing at 125 ml/hr in his right forearm.

5. The surgeon has written to keep E.B.'s stump elevated on pillows for 48 hours; after that, have him lie in a prone position for 15 minutes qid. In teaching E.B. about his care, how would you explain the rationale for these orders?

6. In reviewing E.B.'s medical history, what factor do you notice that may affect the condition of his stump and ultimate rehabilitation potential?

CASE STUDY PROGRESS

You have just returned from a 2-day workshop on guidelines for the care of surgical patients with type 1 DM. You notice that E.B.'s blood glucose has been running between 130 and 180 mg/dl. The sliding-scale insulin intervention does not begin until blood glucose values equal to or greater than 200 mg/dl are reported. You recognize that patients with blood glucose values even slightly above normal suffer from impaired wound healing.

7. Identify four interventions that would facilitate timely healing of E.B.'s stump.

8. What should the postoperative assessment of E.B.'s stump dressing include?

9. On the evening of the first postoperative day, E.B. becomes more awake and begins to C/O pain. He states, "My leg is really hurting; how can it hurt so bad if it's gone?" How would you respond to E.B.'s question?

CASE STUDY PROGRESS

The case manager (CM) is contacted for discharge planning. E.B. will be discharged to an extended care facility for strength training. Once the patient receives his prosthesis, he will receive balance training. After that he will be discharged to his daughter's home. A physical therapy (PT) and occupational therapy (OT) home evaluation should be ordered. Someone from the billing office will explain how the bills will be handled and when.

10. What instructions should be given to E.B.'s daughter concerning safety around the home?

CASE STUDY PROGRESS

E.B. makes a smooth transition from hospital to rehab facility and then to the daughter's home. He was never able to adapt to independent living, so he eventually moved into his daughter's home.

Case Study **41**

Scenario

J.T. has injured his hand at work and is accompanied to the emergency department (ED) by a co-worker. You examine his left hand and find a piece of a drill bit sticking out of the skin between the third and fourth knuckles. There is another puncture site about an inch below and toward the center of the hand. Bleeding is minimal. J.T. is 41 years old, has no significant medical history, and has no known drug allergies (NKDA). He states the accident occurred when a mill at work malfunctioned and knocked his hand onto a rack of drill bits. His last tetanus booster was 3 years ago. It is your job to provide the initial care for J.T.'s injury.

1. You examine J.T.'s hand. What should you include in your initial assessment, and why?

CASE STUDY PROGRESS
You record that J.T.'s fingers are warm with capillary refill in less than 2 seconds. Sensory perception is intact. He is able to flex and extend the distal joints but not the proximal joints of the third and fourth fingers.

2. You notice J.T.'s wedding band and promptly ask him to remove it. Why is this important?

3. J.T. asks you why he can't just pull the bit out and go home. How should you respond to his question?

4. What common diagnostic test will identify fractures and the location of metal fragments in J.T.'s hand?

CASE STUDY PROGRESS

The drill bit is impaled ½ inch below the surface of the skin, and there are no fractures. Because the hand contains so many blood vessels, nerves, ligaments, and tendons, the ED physician decides to consult a surgical hand specialist. A neurologic consult says there is no nerve damage. The surgeon suspects tendon damage and decides to operate immediately.

5. What do you need to do to prepare J.T. for immediate surgery?

6. You record that J.T. has had no food "since 8:00 PM yesterday" and drank "some water" this morning. Based on this information, do you anticipate problems during surgery, and why?

7. Should J.T. be given a tetanus booster before he goes to surgery?

CASE STUDY PROGRESS
The surgeon repairs 2 partially severed tendons and wraps the hand in a large padded dressing. The distal ½ inch of each digit protrudes from the bulky dressing.

8. While in the short-stay recovery area, J.T. asks the nurse why his fingers look yellowish brown. How should she respond to his question?

CASE STUDY PROGRESS
The surgeon tells J.T. that he had to repair tendons in his third and fourth fingers and instructs J.T. that he is not to work. He gives J.T. prescriptions for an antibiotic and an antiinflammatory agent. He instructs J.T. to make an appointment to see him in the surgery clinic in 2 days.

9. What instructions should the nurse in the short-stay area discuss with J.T. and his wife before releasing him?

10. J.T. says, "How in the world is the ice supposed to keep my hand cold with this big bandage on it?" How will the nurse reply?

11. J.T. says, "I'll be able to keep my hand up when I'm awake, but what about when I go to sleep?" What suggestion can the nurse make to help J.T. comply with the instructions?

CASE STUDY PROGRESS

J.T.'s recovery was uncomplicated; he received follow-up (F/U) occupational therapy and regained the full use of his hand.

chapter 4

Gastrointestinal Disorders

Case Study 42

Name _____ Class/Group _____ Date _____
Group Members _____
INSTRUCTIONS All questions apply to this case study. Your responses should be brief and to the point. When asked to provide several answers, list them in order of priority or significance. Do not assume information that is not provided. Please print or write clearly. If your response is not legible, it will be marked as ? and you will need to rewrite it.

Scenario

T.H., a 57-year-old stockbroker, has come to the gastroenterologist for treatment of recurrent mild to severe cramping in his abdomen and blood-streaked stool. You are the RN doing his initial work-up. Your findings include a mildly obese (male-pattern obesity) man who demonstrates moderate guarding of his abdomen with both direct and rebound tenderness, especially in the left lower quadrant (LLQ). His vital signs (VS) are 168/98, 110, 24, 100.4°F, and he is slightly diaphoretic. T.H. reports that he has periodic constipation. He has had previous episodes of abdominal cramping, but this time the pain is getting worse. He has no known drug allergies (NKDA).

Past medical history (PMH) reveals that T.H. has a "sedentary job with lots of emotional moments"; he has smoked a pack of cigarettes a day for 30 years and has had "2 or 3 mixed drinks in the evening" until 2 months ago. He states, "I haven't had anything to drink in 60 days." He denies having regular exercise: "just no time." His diet consists mostly of "white bread, meat, potatoes, and ice cream with fruit and nuts over it." He denies having a history of cardiac or pulmonary problems and no personal history of cancer, although his father and older brother died of colon cancer. He takes no "regular" medications and denies the use of any other drugs.

1. Identify four general health risk problems T.H. exhibits.

2. Identify a key factor in his family history that may have profound implications for his health and present state of mind.

3. Identify three key findings on his physical exam, and indicate their significance.

CASE STUDY PROGRESS

The physician ordered a KUB (x-ray of the kidneys, ureters, bladder), CBC, and complete metabolic profile (CMP). Based on x-ray and lab findings, physical examination, and history, the physician diagnoses T.H. as having acute diverticulitis and discusses an outpatient treatment plan with him.

4. What is diverticulitis? What are the consequences of untreated diverticulitis?

5. While the patient is experiencing the severe crampy pain of acute diverticulitis, what interventions would you perform to help him feel more comfortable?

6. What is the rationale for ordering bed rest and anticholinergics?

7. What classes of medications would be prescribed for someone hospitalized for acute diverticulitis?

CASE STUDY PROGRESS

Metronidazole (Flagyl) and clindamycin (Cleocin) are antibiotics used in conjunction with broad-spectrum penicillin (PCN), cephalosporin, or aminoglycoside to treat diverticulitis. T.H. is being sent home with prescriptions for metronidazole 500 mg PO q6h and amoxicillin-clavulanate (Augmentin) 875 mg PO bid.

8. Given his history, what questions must you ask T.H. before he takes the initial dose of metronidazole? State your rationale.

9. What is a disulfiram reaction?

10. Aside from warning T.H. about the interactions just described, what instructions should you give him regarding his metronidazole prescription?

11. What information would you want to know before starting T.H. on amoxicillin?

12. What are the signs and symptoms (S/S) of an allergic reaction?

13. What will you do if the patient indicates a history of an allergic reaction to PCN?

14. To prevent future episodes of constipation, what dietary changes would the registered dietitian (RD) discuss with T.H. after the acute phase has resolved?

15. You obtain a referral for T.H. to work with an RD on nutritional issues. What measures do you think the RD will discuss with T.H. to avoid recurrent acute diverticulitis?

CASE STUDY PROGRESS

T.H. returns for a check-up 14 days later; all S/S of diverticulitis are gone. He is working on his lifestyle changes and reports he is walking 30 minutes every day. Only 10% to 25% of patients with diverticulitis require any surgery (usually a colectomy). Those who do require surgical treatment often suffer recurrent, uncontrollable diverticulitis.

Case Study **43**

Scenario

T.B. is a 65-year-old retiree who is admitted to your unit from the emergency department (ED). On
arrival you note that he is trembling and nearly doubled over with severe abdominal pain. T.B. indicates
that he has severe pain in the right upper quadrant (RUQ) of his abdomen that radiates through to
his mid-back as a deep, sharp boring pain. He is more comfortable walking or sitting bent forward
rather than lying flat in bed. He admits to having had several similar bouts of abdominal pain in the
last month, but "none as bad as this." He feels nauseated but has not vomited, although he did vomit
a week ago with a similar episode. T.B. experienced an acute onset of pain after eating fish and chips
at a fast-food restaurant earlier today. He is not happy to be in the hospital and is grumpy that his
daughter insisted on taking him to the ED for evaluation.

After orienting him to the room, call light, bed controls, and lights, you perform your physical
assessment. The findings are as follows: he is awake, alert, and oriented (AAO) ×3, and he moves all
extremities well (MAEW). He is restless, is constantly shifting his position, and complains of (C/O)
fatigue. Breath sounds are clear to auscultation (CTA). Heart sounds are clear and crisp, with no murmur
or rub noted and with a regular rate and rhythm (RRR). Abdomen is flat, slightly rigid, and very tender
to palpation throughout, especially in the RUQ; bowel sounds are present. A sharp inspiratory arrest
and exclamation of pain occur with deep palpation of the costal margin in the RUQ (positive Murphy's
sign). He reports light-colored stools for 1 week. The patient voids dark amber urine but denies dysuria.
Skin and sclera are jaundiced. Admission vital signs (VS) are 164/100, 132, 26, 36°C, Sao$_2$ 96% on 2 L
of oxygen by nasal cannula (O$_2$/NC).

1. What structures are located in the RUQ of the abdomen?

2. Which of the above mentioned organs are palpable in the RUQ?

CASE STUDY PROGRESS

T.B.'s abdominal ultrasound (US) demonstrates several retained stones in the common bile duct (CBD)
and a stone-filled gallbladder. T.B. is admitted to your floor, NPO status, and is scheduled to undergo
an endoscopic retrograde cholangiopancreatogram (ERCP) that afternoon. While the patient is sedated,
the ERCP scope is inserted through the mouth and extends past the stomach to the outlet of the CBD,
the ampulla of Vater. Typically this muscle will be cut to widen the opening and outflow of the CBD,
a procedure called a *sphincterotomy*. This allows the bile and stones (cholesterol or pigmented) to
flow out into the small intestine.

3. Given T.B.'s diagnosis, what laboratory values would be important to evaluate?

CASE STUDY PROGRESS

T.B.'s labs show WBC 11.9 thou/cmm, Hgb 14.0 g/dl, Hct 42%, platelets 250 thou/cmm, alanine transaminase (ALT) 200 units/L, aspartate transaminase (AST) 260 units/L, alkaline phosphatase 450 units/L, total bilirubin 4.8 mg/dl, PT 10.5 sec, INR 1.0, amylase 20 units/L, lipase 23 units/L, urinalysis (UA) negative. The patient undergoes the ERCP, and stones and bile are released, but imaging reveals that a stone is still retained within the cystic duct, and multiple stones remain within the gallbladder as well. A surgical consult is obtained, and a laparoscopic cholecystectomy ("lap-choley") is planned.

4. Identify at least four preoperative orders that will likely need to be completed before T.B. goes to surgery.

5. T.B. is medicated with morphine sulfate 2 to 4 mg IV push (IVP) q1-2h. He reports that on a scale of 1 to 10, his pain has decreased from a 10 to a 4 in an hour. What other methods could be used to help T.B.'s pain?

6. What data charted in the assessment are consistent with CBD obstruction?

CASE STUDY PROGRESS

At 2330 T.B. spikes a temperature of 38.6°C (tympanic). His Sao_2 on 2 L O_2/NC is now 90%, so you immediately increase the flow rate to raise his O_2 saturation. You inform the on-call surgeon, and she orders a STAT chest x-ray (CXR) and a broad-spectrum antibiotic—imipenem and cilastatin 500 mg IV q6h (check renal function; this medication must be dose adjusted if patient has renal impairment, or there is an increased risk for seizure).

7. What actions need to be completed before starting the antibiotic?

8. T.B. undergoes a successful laparoscopic cholecystectomy the next morning. An intraoperative cholangiogram shows that the ducts are finally cleared of stones at the conclusion of the surgery. When he returns to the floor, his stomach is soft but quite distended. His wife asks you if anything is wrong. How should you respond?

9. The next day when you remove the tape to change the dressing, you note that the skin is red and blistered underneath. Otherwise he is doing well; he is afebrile, and his vital signs (VS) are 128/72, 80, 16, and Sao_2 of 93% on room air. He even tolerated a light breakfast. To protect the blistered area from further damage, you apply a hydrocolloid dressing, such as DuoDerm, HydraPak, Restore, or Ultec, to the damaged skin. What has T.B. experienced, and what are the benefits of this type of dressing?

10. The rest of the day is uneventful and T.B. is discharged that evening to home. What discharge teaching does T.B. need?

Case Study **44**

Scenario

M.R. is a 56-year-old general contractor who is admitted to your telemetry unit directly from his internist's office with a diagnosis of chest pain. On report, you are informed that he has an intermittent 2-month history of chest tightness with substernal burning that radiates through to the mid-back intermittently, in a stabbing fashion. Symptoms occur after a large meal; with heavy lifting at the construction site; and in the middle of the night when he awakens from sleep with coughing, shortness of breath (SOB), and a foul, bitter taste in his mouth. Recently he has developed nausea, without emesis, worse in the morning or after skipping meals. He complains of "heartburn" 3 or 4 times a day. He takes a couple Rolaids or Tums. He keeps a bottle at home, at the office, and in his truck. Vital signs (VS) at his physician's office were 130/80 lying, 120/72 standing, 100, 20, 98.6°F, Sao_2 92% on room air. A 12-lead ECG showed normal sinus rhythm with a rare premature ventricular contraction (PVC).

1. What are some common causes of chest pain?

2. What mnemonic can you use to help you better evaluate his pain?

3. What other history is important?

CASE STUDY PROGRESS

M.R. indicates that usually the chest pain is relieved with his antacids, but this time they had no effect. A "GI cocktail" consisting of Mylanta and viscous lidocaine given at his physician's office briefly helped decrease symptoms.

4. What tests could be done to determine the source of his problems?

＊**Note:** *If the esophageal mucosa appears normal yet the subjective complaints suggest esophageal acid exposure, the gastroenterologist may place a Bravo 48-hour pH probe within the esophageal wall about 6 cm above the gastroesophageal junction. The probe has a small computer chip that communicates via electronic signal to a receiver unit that is worn like a pager on the belt. If the pH of the esophageal refluxate is over 4.0 a significant amount of time, then it is deemed pathologic.*

CASE STUDY PROGRESS

M.R. has smoked 1 pack of cigarettes a day for the past 35 years, drinks 2 or 3 beers on most nights, and has noticed a 20-pound weight gain over the past 10 years. He feels "so tired and old now." M.R. has dark circles under his eyes and complains of (C/O) daytime fatigue. His wife is even sleeping in another bedroom because he is snoring so loudly. He also reinjured his lower back a month ago at work lifting a pile of boards, so his physician prescribed ibuprofen (Motrin) 800 mg bid or tid for 4 weeks.

5. Which factors in M.R.'s life are likely contributing to his chest pain and nausea? Explain how.

✳ **Note:** *Our innate defense mechanisms against esophageal acid exposure (reflux) include the 3 sequential waves of esophageal muscle contraction that propel the food or liquid down into the stomach; saliva, with its alkaline bicarbonate base that neutralizes the stomach acid on contact; and the lower esophageal sphincter (LES), the circular muscle located at the gastroesophageal junction, which must relax and open to allow food and liquid to pass into the stomach. Inappropriate relaxation of the LES is the primary mechanism by which gastroesophageal reflux disease (GERD) occurs.*

6. What is a hiatal hernia, and what is its role in GERD?

CASE STUDY PROGRESS

M.R. explains that 6 months ago his physician prescribed ranitidine (Zantac) 150 mg PO bid for heart-burn, and that it worked great initially. Now he keeps a bottle of Tums or Rolaids in his truck and at his bedside, in addition to the ranitidine, "because I always seem to need them."

CASE STUDY PROGRESS

M.R.'s 12-lead ECG was normal, and the first set of cardiac enzymes was normal. CBC showed WBC 6.0 thou/cmm, Hgb 15.0 g/dl, Hct 47%, platelets 220 thou/cmm. Complete metabolic panel (CMP) revealed Na 140 mmol/L, K 3.7 mmol/L, BUN 20 mg/dl, creatinine 1.0 mg/dl, lipase 20 unit/L, amylase 18 units/L, PT 12.0 sec, INR 1.0. The chest x-ray (CXR) showed no abnormalities. Room air Sao_2 is 94% and breathing is unlabored. M.R. begins to C/O nausea; as you hand him the emesis basin, he promptly vomits coffee-ground emesis with specks of bright red blood. VS remain stable.

7. What did M.R. vomit?

CASE STUDY PROGRESS

You inform your charge nurse and contact the gastrointestinal (GI) consulting doctor to explain the recent events. The gastroenterologist gives you several orders and states he will be there in 45 minutes. The orders are as follows: NPO status for emergent esophagogastroduodenoscopy (EGD); STAT CBC; O_2 by nasal cannula (NC); titrate oxygen (O_2) to maintain Sao_2 over 90%; type and crossmatch (T&C) 2 units packed RBCs (PRBCs), and hold; start a pantoprazole drip at 8 mg/hr, preceded by an 80-mg bolus over 8 minutes. Insert a nasogastric tube (NGT) and start a gastric lavage with water or saline. Insert 2 large-bore IVs and start normal saline (NS) at 100 ml/hr.

8. Explain the rational for each of the preceding orders and how would you accomplish each.

CASE STUDY PROGRESS

The gastroenterologist finds erosive esophagitis LA Class B, a moderately sized hiatal hernia, diffuse erosive gastritis, and an ulcer in the antrum of the stomach that is oozing blood. The duodenal bulb yielded a normal endoscopic appearance. The endoscopist stopped the bleeding with cautery. Biopsies were obtained of the gastric mucosa to assess for the presence of the infectious agent *Helicobacter pylori*, which is associated with ulcer disease. M.R.'s biopsies are negative for *H. pylori* bacteria, and his bleeding ulcer is attributed to the NSAIDs (i.e., ibuprofen). He is kept NPO until the next morning to allow good hemostasis of the cauterized site. Clear liquids are allowed at breakfast. His hematocrit (Hct) dropped to 32%, but he remained asymptomatic from the mild anemia, and the drop was believed to, in part, reflect the fact that he was dehydrated on admission and the decrease reflected the dilution of the blood from the IV fluids added. Thus he did not receive a transfusion of blood.

M.R. tolerated the liquid diet without any nausea and vomiting (N/V) and is discharged home the next day with the following instructions:

- Advance diet slowly, as tolerated, to mechanical soft.
- Take pantoprazole 40 mg PO q AM on an empty stomach, at least 30 minutes before eating.
- Make a follow-up (F/U) appointment in 6 to 8 weeks with physician (give name and telephone number).
- Stop all aspirin and over-the-counter (OTC) or herbal pain relief medications (ibuprofen, naproxen, etc.).
- Stop or limit alcohol intake and smoking.

9. Why does the patient need to take the pantoprazole (or any proton pump inhibitor [PPI]) first thing in the morning?

10. Lastly, what lifestyle modifications would you recommend for M.R. on discharge to prevent acid reflux?

Case Study **45**

Name _____ Class/Group _____ Date _____
Group Members _____

INSTRUCTIONS All questions apply to this case study. Your responses should be brief and to the point. When asked to provide several answers, list them in order of priority or significance. Do not assume information that is not provided. Please print or write clearly. If your response is not legible, it will be marked as ? and you will need to rewrite it.

Scenario

While you are working as a nurse on a gastrointestinal/genitourinary (GI/GU) floor, you receive a call from your affiliate outpatient clinic notifying you of a direct admission, ETA (estimated time of arrival) 60 minutes. She gives you the following information: A.G. is an 87-year-old woman with a 3-day history of intermittent abdominal pain, abdominal bloating, and nausea and vomiting (N/V). A.G. moved from Italy to join her grandson and his family only 2 months ago, and she speaks little English. All information was obtained through her grandson. Past medical history (PMH) includes colectomy for colon cancer 6 years ago and ventral hernia repair 2 years ago. She has no history of coronary artery disease (CAD), diabetes mellitus (DM), or pulmonary disease. She takes only ibuprofen occasionally for mild arthritis. Allergies include sulfa drugs and meperidine. A.G.'s tentative diagnosis is small bowel obstruction (SBO) secondary to adhesions. A.G. is being admitted to your floor for diagnostic work-up. Her vital signs (VS) are stable, she has an IV of $D_5\frac{1}{2}NS$ with 20 mEq KCl at 100 ml/hr, and 3 L oxygen by nasal cannula (O_2/NC).

1. Based on the nurse's report, what signs of bowel obstruction did A.G. manifest?

2. Are there other signs and symptoms (S/S) that you should observe for while A.G. is in your care?

3. A.G. and her grandson arrive on your unit. You admit A.G. to her room and introduce yourself as her nurse. As her grandson interprets for her, she pats your hand. You know that you need to complete a physical examination and take a history. What will you do first?

4. The grandson, an attorney, tells you elderly Italian women are extremely modest and may not answer questions completely. How might you gather information in this case?

5. What key questions must you ask this patient while you have the use of an interpreter?

6. How would the description of A.G.'s pain differ if she has a small versus large bowel obstruction?

7. With some difficulty, you insert a nasogastric tube (NGT) into A.G. and connect it to intermittent low wall suction (LWS). How will you check for placement of the NGT?

8. List, in order, the structures through which the NGT must pass as it is inserted.

9. What comfort measures are important for A.G. while she has an NGT?

10. You note that A.G.'s NGT has not drained in the last 3 hours. What can you do to facilitate drainage?

11. The NGT suddenly drains 575 ml; then it slows down to about 250 ml over 2 hours. Is this an expected amount?

12. You enter A.G.'s room to initiate your shift assessment. A.G. has been hospitalized 3 days, and her abdomen seems to be more distended than yesterday. How would you determine whether A.G.'s abdominal distention has changed?

CASE STUDY PROGRESS

After 3 days of NGT suction, A.G.'s symptoms are unrelieved. She reports continued nausea, cramps, and sometimes strong abdominal pain; her hand grips are weaker; and she seems to be increasingly lethargic. You look up her latest laboratory values and compare them with the admission data. Her sodium (Na) has changed from 136 to 130 mmol/L, potassium (K) has changed from 3.7 to 2.5 mmol/L, chloride (Cl) from 108 to 97 mmol/L, carbon dioxide (CO_2) from 25 to 31 mmol/L, BUN from 19 to 38 mg/dl, creatinine from 1 to 2.2 mg/dl, glucose from 126 to 65 mg/dl, albumin from 3.0 to 2.1 g/dl, and protein from 6.8 to 4.9 g/dl.

13. Which lab values are of concern to you? Why?

14. What measures do you anticipate to correct each of the imbalances described in question 13?

CASE STUDY PROGRESS

In view of A.G.'s continued slow deterioration, the surgeon met with the patient and her family and they agreed to surgery. The surgeon released an 18-inch section of proximal ileum that had been constricted by adhesions. Several areas looked ischemic, so these were excised, and an end-to-end anastomosis was done. A.G. tolerated the procedure well and recovered rapidly from the anesthesia in the postanesthesia care unit (PACU). Once on the unit, her recovery was slow but steady. A.G. went home in the care of her grandson and his wife on the seventh postoperative day. Discharge plans included home health nurse, home health aide, in-home physical therapy, and dietitian consult. The grandson was included in any plans.

Case Study **46**

Name _____ Class/Group _____ Date _____
Group Members _____
INSTRUCTIONS All questions apply to this case study. Your responses should be brief and to the point. When asked
to provide several answers, list them in order of priority or significance. Do not assume information that is not provided.
Please print or write clearly. If your response is not legible, it will be marked as ? and you will need to rewrite it.

Scenario

P.M., a 24-year-old house painter, has been too ill to work for the past 3 days. When he arrives at your outpatient clinic, he seems an alert but acutely ill young man of average build, with a deep tan over exposed
areas of skin. He reports headaches, severe myalgia, a low-grade fever, cough, anorexia, and nausea and
vomiting (N/V), especially after eating any fatty food. P.M. describes vague abdominal pain that started
about the same time as the other problems. His past medical history (PMH) reveals he has no health problems, is a nonsmoker, and drinks a "few" beers each evening to relax. Vital signs (VS) are 128/84, 88, 26,
100.6°F; awake, alert, and oriented (AAO) ×3; moves all extremities well (MAEW) except for aching pain
in his muscles; very slight scleral jaundice present; heart tones clear and without adventitious sounds;
bowel sounds clear throughout abdomen and pelvis; abdomen soft and palpable without distinct masses.
You note moderate hepatomegaly measured at the midclavicular line; liver edge is easily palpated and
tender to palpation. P.M. mentions that his urine has been getting darker over the past 2 days.

P.M. is manifesting the key signs of hepatitis. Lab work is sent for identification of his precise
problem. Results are Na 140 mmol/L, K 3.9 mmol/L, Cl 102 mmol/L, CO_2 26 mmol/L, BUN 10 mg/dl,
creatinine 1.0 mg/dl, platelets 86 thou/cmm, direct bilirubin 1.6 mg/dl, total bilirubin 2.3 mg/dl, albumin
3.8 g/dl, total protein 6.2 g/dl, alanine aminotransferase (ALT) 66 units/L, aspartate aminotransferase
(AST) 52 units/L, lactate dehydrogenase (LDH) 205 units/L, alkaline phosphatase 176 units/L, PT 12 sec,
INR 1.06, PTT 32 sec. Urine urobilinogen is 1.6 IU/L, albuminuria 160 mg/dl, positive for bilirubinuria,
positive for anti-HAV (hepatitis A virus) IgM.

1. Which key diagnostic tests will determine exactly what type of hepatitis is present?

2. A CBC, BMP, LFT, and PT/PTT were drawn. Which of the lab values listed above
specifically indicates liver disease?

3. List three drugs that can cause increased ALT levels.

4. Considering that the basic pathology of hepatitis involves inflammation, degeneration, and regeneration of the hepatocyte, what type of diet will you strongly encourage P.M. to follow?

5. Differentiate between hepatitis A, B, and C on the basis of the mode of transmission and prevention.

6. Name three major activities that can be done in a community to prevent the spread of hepatitis (all types).

7. In P.M.'s case, the IgM class anti-HAV antibody is positive. This result indicates that P.M. is infected with hepatitis A and is in the acute or early convalescent period of the disease. Is this disease contagious? What precaution would you take?

8. Pruritus is usually associated with jaundice. What will you do to ease this problem for P.M.?

9. How would you explain to P.M. the likely progression of his disease? (This approach requires not only knowledge of disease and its progression but an ability to figure out P.M.'s thought processes.)

10. P.M. is living at home with his parents and 4 younger siblings. The youngest is 4 years old. His parents ask how to prevent the rest of the family from getting hepatitis. What specific instructions will you give? How will you know that these instructions are understood?

11. Given P.M.'s lifestyle, what specific patient teaching points must you emphasize?

Case Study **47**

Name _____ Class/Group _____ Date _____
Group Members _____

INSTRUCTIONS All questions apply to this case study. Your responses should be brief and to the point. When asked to provide several answers, list them in order of priority or significance. Do not assume information that is not provided. Please print or write clearly. If your response is not legible, it will be marked as ? and you will need to rewrite it.

Scenario

John Doe no. 6, approximately 50 years old, is admitted to your floor from the emergency department (ED). He is lethargic, has a cachectic appearance, does not follow commands consistently, and is mildly combative when aroused. He smells strongly of alcohol (ETOH) and has a notably distended abdomen and edematous lower extremities.

This man was sent to the ED by local police, who found him lying unresponsive along a rural road. He was aroused somewhat in the ED. Examination and x-ray studies are negative for any injury, and he is admitted to your unit for observation. He has no ID and is not awake or coherent enough to give any history or to answer questions. Admitting orders are admit to the medical floor with rule out (R/O) hepatic encephalopathy with acute ETOH intoxication; IV $D_5\frac{1}{2}NS$ with 20 mEq KCl at 75 ml/hr; add 1 ampule multivitamins (MVI) to 1 L of IV fluid (IVF) per day; hook up nasogastric tube (NGT) to low wall suction (LWS); Foley catheter to down drain (DD); elevate head of bed (HOB) at 30 to 45 degrees at all times; lactulose 45 ml PO qid until 3 soft stools; abdominal ultrasound (US) in AM; CBC with differential, basic metabolic panel (BMP), liver function tests (LFTs), PT/PTT, NH_3 now and in AM; soft restraints prn; vitamin K 10 mg/day IV or PO ×3 doses; thiamine 100 mg/day IM; folic acid 5 mg/day IM; pyridoxine 100 mg/day PO. Once patient is able to take things by mouth, he should be given a low-protein diet and eat with assistance only. Call house officer (HO) for any sign of gastrointestinal (GI) bleed; delirium tremens (DTs); systolic blood pressure (SBP) over 140 or less than 100 mm Hg; or diastolic BP (DBP) less than 50 mm Hg; or pulse over 120 beats/min.

1. Which of the preceding orders must be done by the RN? By the aide? By the clerk?

2. The lab work drawn in the ED has come back. The blood alcohol level (BAL) is 320 mg/dl, and the blood ammonia (NH_3) level is 155 mcg/dl. What do these values indicate?

CASE STUDY PROGRESS

While you are getting John Doe settled, you continue your assessment. Neurologic findings are PERRL (*Pupils Equal, Round, Reactive to Light*), MAEW, patient is sluggish, pulling away during assessment, follows commands sporadically. Cerebrovascular findings are pulse regular but tachycardic without adventitious sounds. All peripheral pulses palpable, with 3+ bilateral, 3+ pitting edema in lower extremities. John Doe is given an IV of $D_5\frac{1}{2}NS$ with 1 ampule MVI and 20 mEq KCl/L at 75 ml/hr in left forearm. Respiratory assessment reveals breath sounds decreased to all lobes, no adventitious sounds audible, patient not cooperating with cough and deep breathing (C&DB), and Sao_2 at 90% on room air. GI findings are tongue and gums are beefy red and swollen, abdomen is enlarged and protuberant, girth is 141 cm, and abdominal skin is taut and slightly tender to palpation. His NGT is patent, bowel sounds positive with NGT clamped. Genitourinary (GU) assessment reveals Foley to DD with 75 ml dark amber urine since admission (2 hours). Skin is pale on his torso and lower extremities (LEs), heavily sunburned on his upper extremities (UEs) and head. Skin appears thin and dry. Numerous spider angiomas are found on the upper abdomen with several dilated veins across abdomen. Vital signs (VS) are 120/60, 104, 32, 37.3°C. His protein is 5.2 g/dl, and albumin is 2.1 g/dl. A toxicology screen and electrolytes have been drawn.

3. What is the significance of the spider angiomas, dilated abdominal veins, peripheral edema, and distended abdomen?

4. How would you further assess the distended abdomen, and what is the clinical name for your findings?

5. What is your concern about John Doe's nutritional status? What are your objective findings?

6. Why isn't John Doe on a high–protein diet?

7. How might you respond to fellow staff nurses' remarks, "Why are we wasting time with this 'wino'? He isn't worth the time or money. Why don't they let him die?"

8. A nursing problem relative to John Doe's care is risk for injury. Ensuring safety is a critical part of the nursing role. Identify two areas of injury risk, and specify actions you will take to ensure his safety.

9. What are the signs and symptoms (S/S) of DTs?

10. Falls are particularly dangerous for someone in this patient's situation. Why?

CASE STUDY PROGRESS

During detoxification, most alcoholics exhibit a variety of cognitive deficits, including reduced verbal skills, learning difficulty, slowing of responses, and visual perceptual problems. These deficits may be permanent or they may improve with abstinence over time. A psychologist can evaluate John Doe for mental decline associated with alcohol abuse and dependence, including alcoholic dementia, or Korsakoff's psychosis.

11. What are alcoholic dementia and Korsakoff's psychosis?

CASE STUDY PROGRESS

John Doe survives a rocky course of hepatic encephalopathy and near-renal failure. After 27 days, including a week in the ICU, he is discharged to a drug and alcohol rehabilitation facility. He is employed as a longshoreman; fortunately, his insurance covers his month of in-house intense rehabilitation.

Case Study **48**

Name _____ Class/Group _____ Date _____
Group Members _____
INSTRUCTIONS All questions apply to this case study. Your responses should be brief and to the point. When asked
to provide several answers, list them in order of priority or significance. Do not assume information that is not provided.
Please print or write clearly. If your response is not legible, it will be marked as ? and you will need to rewrite it.

Scenario

C.W., a 36-year-old woman, was admitted several days ago with a diagnosis of recurrent inflammatory bowel disease (IBD) and possible small bowel obstruction (SBO). C.W. is married, and her husband and 11-year-old son are supportive, but she has no extended family in-state. She has had IBD for 15 years and has been taking mesalamine (Asacol) for 15 years and prednisone 40 mg/day for the past 5 years. She is very thin; at 5'2" she weighs 86 pounds and has lost 40 pounds over the past 10 years. She has an average of 5 to 10 loose stools per day. C.W.'s life has gradually become dominated by her disease (anorexia; lactase deficiency; profound fatigue; frequent nausea and diarrhea; frequent hospitalizations for dehydration; and recurring, crippling abdominal pain that often strikes unexpectedly). The pain is incapacitating and relieved only by a small dose of diazepam (Valium), Pedialyte, and total bed rest. She confides in you that sexual activity is difficult: "It always causes diarrhea, nausea, and lots of pain. It's difficult for both of us." She is so weak she cannot stand without help. You write complete bed rest (CBR) with side rails up on the Kardex. (You also make a mental note of the probability that she has osteoporosis secondary to long-term steroid use.)

1. Identify six priority problems for C.W.

2. You enter C.W.'s room and note that she has been crying. You ask what's wrong, and she explains that the nurse who admitted her to the hospital the last time said, "Welcome to death row!" C.W. says that she is knowledgeable about her condition, but she still can't seem to shake that "death row" feeling. She was afraid to come to the hospital this time. What can you do to help this woman?

CASE STUDY PROGRESS

C.W. states, "Treat me with respect, and as a person, not a disease. Act like I have the right and intelligence to understand my condition. Recognize that I probably know what I'm talking about when I refuse a delicious milkshake. When I'm either NPO or nauseated, please don't pop popcorn where I can smell it! It's pure torture!"

3. Considering C.W.'s weakness, chronic diarrhea, and lower-than-desired body weight, what interventions should minimize skin breakdown?

CASE STUDY PROGRESS

C.W.'s condition deteriorates on the third day after admission; she experiences intractable abdominal pain and unrelenting nausea and vomiting (N/V). C.W. is taken to the operating room (OR) for probable SBO and is readmitted to your unit from the postanesthesia care unit (PACU). During surgery, 38 inches of her small bowel were found to be severely stenosed with 2 areas of visible perforation. Much of the remaining bowel is severely inflamed and friable. A total of 5 feet of distal ileum and 2 feet of colon have been removed, and a temporary ileostomy was established. She has a Jackson-Pratt (JP) drain to bulb suction in her right lower quadrant (RLQ), and her wound was packed and left open. She has two peripheral IVs, a nasogastric tube (NGT), and a Foley catheter. Her vital signs (VS) are 112/72, 86, 24, 100.8° F (tympanic).

�֍ **4.** You begin a thorough postoperative assessment of C.W.'s abdomen. What does your assessment include? List these steps in the order in which the assessment should be completed.

5. A nursing student enters C.W.'s room and auscultates her abdomen. She looks at you and excitedly announces that she hears good bowel sounds. You take the opportunity to teach her the proper method of auscultating bowel sounds on a patient who has NGT to continuous low wall suction (LWS). How would you correct her error?

CASE STUDY PROGRESS

The nursing student follows your advice and listens again. She says "You're right, I didn't hear a thing." You tell her that she can impress her classmates while educating them in the correct technique.

6. C.W. is 4 days postop. During the routine dressing change, you note a small pool of yellow-green drainage in the deepest part of the wound. You realize the physician will want a wound culture. How will you culture C.W.'s wound?

7. You obtain a wound culture, complete the dressing change, obtain a full set of VS, note a temperature of 100.4°F, and assess increased tenderness in C.W.'s abdomen. You call to notify the physician and ask for additional orders. What orders do you anticipate?

8. What information do you need to send to the lab with the wound culture specimen?

9. The physician calls back and asks you to describe C.W.'s wound. What key aspects of the wound should be included?

10. The physician asks you how C.W.'s stoma and drainage look. What should a healthy stoma and usual drainage look like?

11. Will any aspect of C.W.'s history significantly affect the wound healing process? How?

12. With a fairly significant wound infection developing, why is C.W.'s temperature relatively low?

13. The physician tells you that she will be over to examine C.W. As you tell C.W. that her doctor is coming to talk to her, C.W. says that she feels something wet running down her side. You find some leakage of intestinal drainage onto the skin. What should you do?

CASE STUDY PROGRESS

You change the ileostomy appliance before the physician arrives. C.W. is evaluated, and it is determined that she should return to surgery for exploratory laparotomy.

Case Study **49**

Name _____ Class/Group _____ Date _____
Group Members _____
INSTRUCTIONS All questions apply to this case study. Your responses should be brief and to the point. When asked to provide several answers, list them in order of priority or significance. Do not assume information that is not provided. Please print or write clearly. If your response is not legible, it will be marked as ? and you will need to rewrite it.

Scenario (Continuation of Case Study 48)

C.W. is a 36-year-old woman admitted 7 days ago for inflammatory bowel disease (IBD) with small bowel obstruction (SBO). She underwent surgery 3 days after admission for a colectomy and ileostomy. She developed peritonitis and 4 days later returned to the operating room (OR) for an exploratory laparotomy, which revealed another area of perforated bowel, generalized peritonitis, and a fistula tract to the abdominal surface. Another 12 inches of ileum were resected (total of 7 feet of ileum and 2 feet of colon). The peritoneal cavity was irrigated with normal saline (NS), and 3 drainage tubes were placed: a Jackson-Pratt (JP) drain to bulb suction, a rubber catheter to irrigate the wound bed with NS, and a sump drain to remove the irrigation. The initial JP drain remains in place. A right subclavian triple-lumen catheter was inserted.

1. C.W. returns from postanesthesia recovery unit (PACU) on your shift. What do you do when her bed is rolled into her room?

2. You pull the covers back to inspect the abdominal dressing and find that the original surgical dressing is saturated with fresh bloody drainage. What should you do?

3. C.W. has a total of 4 tubes in her abdomen, as well as a nasogastric tube (NGT). What information do you want to know about each tube?

✳**Note:** *For safety, all tubes should be clearly labeled.*

4. The sump irrigation fluid bag is nearly empty. You close the roller clamp, thread the IV tubing through the infusion pump, check the irrigation catheter connection site to make certain it is snug, and then discover that the nearly empty liter bag infusing into C.W.'s abdomen is D_5W, not NS. Does this require any action? If so, give rationale for actions, and explain the overall situation.

CASE STUDY PROGRESS

The physician arrives on the unit and removes C.W.'s surgical dressing. There is a small "bleeder" at the edge of the incision, so the physician calls for a suture and ties off the bleeder. You take the opportunity to ask her about a morphine patient-controlled analgesia (PCA) pump for C.W., and the physician says she will write the orders right away.

5. Postoperative pain will be a problem for C.W. after the anesthesia wears off. How do you plan to address this?

6. Pharmacy delivers C.W.'s first bag of total parenteral nutrition (TPN). The physician has instructed you to start the TPN at a rate of 60 ml/hr and decrease the maintenance IV rate by the same amount. What is the purpose of this order?

7. The physician did not specifically order glucose monitoring, but you know that it should be initiated. You plan to conduct a fingerstick blood test every 2 hours for the first several hours. What is your rationale?

8. C.W.'s blood glucose increased temporarily, but by the next day it dropped to an average of 70 to 80 mg/dl and has remained there for 2 days. Her VS are stable, but her abdominal wound shows no signs of healing. She has lost 1 kg over the past 3 days. What do these data mean?

CASE STUDY PROGRESS

You discuss your concerns with C.W.'s physician, and she agrees to request a consult from a registered dietitian (RD). After gathering data and making several calculations, the RD makes recommendations to the attending physician. The TPN orders are adjusted, C.W. begins to gain weight slowly, and her wound shows signs of healing. Nutritional problems in clinical populations can be complex and often require special attention.

9. You and a co-worker read the following in C.W.'s progress notes: "Wound healing by secondary closure. Formation of granular tissue with epithelialization noted around edges. Have requested dietitian to consult on ongoing basis. Will continue to follow." Your co-worker turns to you and asks whether you know what that means. How would you explain?

10. Both of you start to discuss what specific digestive difficulties C.W. is likely to face in the future. What problems might C.W. be prone to develop after having so much of her bowel removed?

11. The RD consults with C.W. about dietary needs. You attend the session so that you will be able to reinforce the information. What basic information is the RD likely to discuss with C.W.?

12. After 3 days of dressing changes, C.W.'s skin is irritated, and a small skin tear has appeared where tape was removed. How can you minimize this type of skin breakdown and help this area heal?

13. What specifics of ostomy teaching do you plan to do?

CASE STUDY PROGRESS

C.W. successfully battled peritonitis. Gradually, tubes were removed as she grew stronger with TPN and time. C.W. learned how to change her ostomy appliance and was discharged home.

Case Study **50**

Scenario

You are a nurse working on a surgical unit and take the following report from the RN in the emergency department (ED). "We are sending you a direct admit with R/O SBO [rule out small bowel obstruction] and/or food blockage. Dr. N., the GI [gastrointestinal] doctor is on his way in to see the patient. D.S. is a 78-year-old obese man with complaints of [C/O] sudden onset of severe abdominal cramping, distention, and nausea and vomiting [N/V]; he denies passing of flatus or stool within the past 12 hours. PMH [past medical history] includes congestive heart failure [CHF], hypertension [HTN], colon cancer, ulcerative colitis. He underwent a total colectomy 16 years ago and had an enterocutaneous fistula 12 years ago. Lab samples have been drawn, and the results will be sent to your floor. We started an IV and placed a nasogastric tube [NGT]. His vital signs [VS] are 143/76, 82, 26 and slightly labored, and 38.4°C. He is on his way up."

1. Given that D.S. had a total colectomy, you know he has an ileostomy. What is the difference between a colostomy and ileostomy, where would the stoma be located, and what type of drainage should you expect from each?

CASE STUDY PROGRESS

After D.S. is settled into his room, the NGT and IV are functioning well, and he receives pain medication, you begin your admission assessment. His abdomen is extremely large, firm to touch, with multiple scars and an ileostomy pouching system in his right lower quadrant (RLQ).

2. What are the more common complications of an ileostomy?

3. How would you determine whether the stoma is healthy?

4. What stoma changes would you report to the physician immediately?

5. Why are transparent ostomy pouches recommended postop or when patients are hospitalized?

6. Will the stoma present visual clues of blockage or obstruction?

7. Why is a peristomal hernia a problem?

CASE STUDY PROGRESS

D.S. continues to C/O abdominal pain and cramping and becomes increasingly restless. You notice that the abdomen behind and around his stoma and pouch appears larger when compared with the other side of his abdomen.

8. How would you assess for a possible hernia?

CASE STUDY PROGRESS

You note that the ostomy pouch has liquid brown effluent along the lateral edge of the wafer. You check to see that the pouch is properly attached to the wafer and discover that stool is indeed leaking from under the barrier. D.S. apologizes for not bringing any supplies with him, stating "my ostomy nurse told me to always carry extra supplies for times like this."

CASE STUDY PROGRESS

D.S. does not remember what size he needs, but you note he is wearing a 2-piece system with a plastic ring-flange that attaches somewhat like a Tupperware seal.

9. How will you determine the correct pouching size and system?

CASE STUDY PROGRESS

You have finished with your general head-to-toe assessment and order the appropriate pouching products for D.S. You have already taken clean towels, washcloths, and underpads into his room, along with a hamper to receive dirty, used laundry. You gather scissors, skin-prep, and adhesive remover to assist with the pouching change.

❈ **10.** As you return to his room, you review the steps for changing an ostomy pouch. What are the steps you will need to follow?

CASE STUDY PROGRESS

You have gathered all needed supplies, and D.S. is as comfortable as possible. You begin the pouching change. Using the adhesive remover, with the push-pull method, you gently remove the wafer. As you lift the wafer, you note that the peristomal skin has severe erythema directly encircling the stoma. There is denudation (partial-thickness breakdown) at the medial stoma-skin edge.

11. How should the skin around the stoma look?

12. Generally there are four different causes of erythema or skin breakdown. Identify two.

Case Study **51**

Scenario

B.K. is a 63-year-old woman who is admitted to the medical-surgical floor from the emergency department (ED) with nausea and vomiting (N/V) and epigastric and left upper quadrant (LUQ) abdominal pain that is severe, sharp, and boring and radiates through to her mid-back. The pain started 24 hours ago and awoke her in the middle of the night. B.K. is a divorced, retired sales manager who smokes a half-pack of cigarettes daily. The ED nurse reports that B.K. is anxious and demanding. Her vital signs (VS) are as follows: 100/70, 97, 30, 100.2°F (tympanic), Sao$_2$ 88% on room air and 92% on 2 L of oxygen by nasal cannula (O$_2$/NC). She is in normal sinus rhythm (NSR). She will be admitted under the on-duty hospitalist because she has no primary care provider (PCP) and hasn't seen a physician "in years."

The ED nurse giving you the report states that the admitting diagnosis is acute pancreatitis of unknown etiology. Unfortunately the CT scanner is down and won't be fixed until morning. However, an ultrasound (US) of the abdomen was performed, and "no cholelithiasis, gallbladder wall thickening, or choledocholithiasis was seen. The pancreas was not well visualized due to overlying bowel gas." Admitting labs include lipase 3000 units/L, amylase 2000 units/L, alkaline phosphatase 350 units/L, alanine transaminase (ALT) 90 units/L, aspartate transaminase (AST) 150 units/L, total bilirubin 2.0 mg/dl, albumin 3.0 g/dl, BUN 26 mg/dl, creatinine 1.0 mg/dl, WBC 17.5 thou/cmm, and Hct 36%. A clean-catch urine sample was just sent to the lab, but the urine was dark.

1. What are the possible causes of pancreatitis?

2. If a CT scan is planned for the morning, what orders would you expect?

3. What other information do you need from this nurse before you assume responsibility for the patient?

4. What approach would you use to obtain a psychosocial history and complete your physical assessment?

CASE STUDY PROGRESS

You complete your assessment and note the following abnormalities: B.K. is restless and lying on her right side in a semifetal position. Cerebrovascular findings are skin is cool, diaphoretic, and pale with poor skin turgor; mucous membranes are dry. Heart rate is regular but tachycardic, without murmurs or rubs. Peripheral pulses are faintly palpable in 4 extremities. Respirations are rapid but unlabored on 2 L O_2/NC with Sao_2 90%. Breath sounds absent in lower left lobe (LLL) posteriorly, otherwise clear to auscultation (CTA) throughout. She complains of (C/O) nausea and is having dry heaves. Bowel sounds are hypoactive. Abdomen is distended, firm, and exquisitely tender in a diffuse fashion to light palpation, with guarding noted.

5. Which labs are the most important to monitor in acute pancreatitis? Why are they significant?

6. What do the BUN and creatinine tell you about her renal function and volume status?

7. Why are the WBCs elevated?

8. B.K. turns on her call light. She C/O thirst and demands something to drink. Her orders indicate "NPO, except sips and chips." How should you respond? What nursing action would help her complaints?

9. During your physical exam, you noted "respirations rapid but unlabored on 2 L O_2/NC with Sao_2 90%. Breath sounds absent in LLL posteriorly, otherwise clear to auscultation throughout." The admission chest x-ray (CXR) report reads, "small pleural effusion in the LLL." Identify three actions you could initiate to help correct this situation.

CASE STUDY PROGRESS

B.K. eventually falls asleep and seems to be sleeping peacefully. Several hours later you hear an alarm on her pulse oximeter and enter her room to investigate. You find B.K. moaning softly; her oximeter reads 87%.

✿ **10.** What should you do next?

11. Your assessment findings are as follows: lung sounds absent in the LLL and very diminished in the right lower lobe (RLL). You percuss a dull thud over the left middle lobe (LML) and LLL up to the scapula tip. On percussion, you hear resonance over the entire right lung and left upper lobe (LUL). What is the significance of your findings?

✿ **12.** What actions should you take next?

CASE STUDY PROGRESS

The physician orders a STAT CXR, which shows a significant pleural effusion developing in the LLL, with extension into the RLL.

13. Based on the evolving pleural effusion with evidence of decompensation (hypoxia) by the patient, what treatment would the physician likely pursue, and what preparations would you be responsible for?

CASE STUDY PROGRESS

The physician removed 200 ml of slightly cloudy serous fluid. Antibiotics were adjusted to provide broad-spectrum coverage for an upper respiratory tract infection (URI) until culture and sensitivity (C&S) results return. An abdominal CT scan is completed and shows "a moderately severe pancreatitis, but no local fluid collection or pseudocysts. No ileus or evidence of neoplasia was noted." It is now 72 hours after B.K.'s admission, and her labs show improvement: BUN 9.0 mg/dl and creatinine 1.0 mg/dl. She has adequate urinary output. Her IV fluids are decreased to 75 ml/hr. Amylase and lipase are also resolving nicely, so the physician advances B.K.'s diet to full liquids.

14. How would you know if the advancement in diet weren't tolerated?

15. If B.K. does not tolerate the advancement in diet, what physiologic need should staff be prepared to address at 72 hours?

CASE STUDY PROGRESS

The afternoon of the third day of B.K.'s hospitalization, she becomes agitated with unintentional tremors, some disorientation, and auditory hallucinations. Her pulse and blood pressure (BP) are elevated, although her pain has not increased, nor has the pain medication schedule changed. B.K. has had no visitors since being admitted.

16. What is B.K. most likely experiencing, and what actions should you take?

CASE STUDY PROGRESS

You contact the physician with your observations, and he orders scheduled chlordiazepoxide and a social work consult to evaluate and treat possible alcohol abuse. B.K. eventually admits to drinking "3 or 4 scotch-on-the-rocks" daily, a good "4 fingers deep each." You also discover that B.K. is estranged from her family because of her drinking.

Three days later, B.K. is tolerating clear liquids, and her pain is controlled with oral pain medications. The physician advances her diet to "low-fat/low-cholesterol" and writes orders to discharge that evening if she tolerates the advancement in diet, which she does.

17. What should you include in your discharge teaching with B.K.?

chapter 5

Genitourinary Disorders

Case Study **52**

Scenario

You are working in an extended care facility (ECF) when M.Z.'s daughter brings her mother in for a
week stay while she goes on vacation. M.Z. is an 89-year-old widow with a 4-day history of dysuria,
back pain, incontinence, severe mental confusion, and loose stools. Her physician discontinued her
hormone replacement therapy (HRT) 1 month ago. Her most current vital signs (VS) are 118/60, 88,
18, 99.4°F.

The medical director ordered several lab tests on admission. The results were as follows: WBC 11
thou/cmm, complete metabolic panel (CMP) within normal limits (WNL). Postvoid catheterization
yielded 100 ml, and urinalysis (UA) showed WBC 100+/HPF (high-powered field), RBC 3 to 6/HPF,
bacteria rare. The urinary culture and sensitivity (C&S) results were as follows: *Escherichia coli*, more
than 100,000 colonies, sensitive to ciprofloxacin, trimethoprim-sulfamethoxazole, and nitrofurantoin.

1. The medical director makes rounds and writes orders to start an IV of D_5.25NS at
75 ml/hr and insert a Foley to down drain (DD). Because M.Z. is unable to take oral
meds, the medical director ordered ciprofloxacin 200 mg bid IV piggyback (IVPB). Is the
type of fluid and rate appropriate for M.Z.'s age and condition? Explain.

2. What signs and symptoms (S/S) will you look for in a patient receiving IV ciprofloxacin?

3. You enter the room to start the IV and insert the Foley catheter but find the aide has taken the patient to the bathroom for a bowel movement (BM). You open the door to observe the patient wiping herself from back to front. You realize this is a teaching moment and take the aide aside and instruct her. What is the association between M.Z.'s urinary tract infection (UTI) and the organism found in her urine culture?

4. As you insert the Foley catheter, you note the introitus is red and dry; no vaginal discharge is noted. You inform the managing physician that M.Z. has atrophic vaginitis and get an order for vaginal estrogen replacement (estradiol [Estrace cream or an Estrace vaginal ring]). M.Z.'s daughter will need to be instructed how to insert the cream or ring for her mother. Outline your teaching plan.

5. What should you instruct the daughter to look for and report to M.Z.'s physician?

6. The aide comes to you to report that M.Z. is picking at her IV and asks if she can apply wrist restraints. How should you respond?

7. If M.Z. develops diarrhea, what special instructions should you give the nursing assistant assigned to give basic care to M.Z.?

8. You are the nurse assigned to M.Z.'s care. You notice that the nursing assistant emptying the gravity drain is not wearing personal protection devices. You also observe that the spout of the drainage bag is contaminated during the process. What issues need to be considered in protecting M.Z.'s safety? Describe your actions in working with the nursing assistant.

9. The nursing assistant reports that M.Z.'s 8-hour intake is 520 ml and the output is 140 ml. Is this significant? Identify two possible reasons that could account for the difference and explain how you would assess each.

10. M.Z. has completed her antibiotic therapy, her mental status has cleared, and she is ready for discharge. What instructions should you discuss with the daughter?

Case Study **53**

Name _____ Class/Group_____Date _____
Group Members _____
INSTRUCTIONS All questions apply to this case study. Your responses should be brief and to the point. When asked
to provide several answers, list them in order of priority or significance. Do not assume information that is not provided.
Please print or write clearly. If your response is not legible, it will be marked as ? and you will need to rewrite it.

Scenario

You are working in the emergency department (ED) when M.B., a 72-year-old man, enters with a chief
complaint (C/C) of inability to void. His initial vital signs (VS) are 168/92, 70, 20, 98.2°F.

1. Are M.B.'s VS appropriate for a man his age? If not, offer a rational for the abnormal readings.

CASE STUDY PROGRESS
While you are taking M.B.'s history, he tells you he is generally in good health and leads an active life.
His current medications include finasteride (Proscar) 5 mg/day and vitamin supplements. He reports
that he has been unable to void for 12 hours and is very uncomfortable. He asks you to help him.

2. Given M.B.'s C/C, what would you expect to find during your initial assessment?

3. What are your priorities for this patient?

4. After examining M.B., the ED physician asks you to insert an indwelling urethral coudé Foley catheter. What should you include in M.B.'s teaching before placing the Foley?

5. After 2 unsuccessful attempts to advance the catheter into the bladder, you stop. What is your next intervention? Why?

6. The ED physician successfully inserts the indwelling catheter and writes orders to discharge M.B. with instructions to see his primary care provider (PCP) the following day. It is your responsibility to give discharge instructions. Outline your care plan.

Case Study **54**

Name _____ Class/Group _____ Date _____

Group Members _____

INSTRUCTIONS All questions apply to this case study. Your responses should be brief and to the point. When asked to provide several answers, list them in order of priority or significance. Do not assume information that is not provided. Please print or write clearly. If your response is not legible, it will be marked as ? and you will need to rewrite it.

Scenario

You are working on a postoperative surgical floor and are assigned to A.T., a 65-year-old woman with a 30-year smoking history who has recently had a radical cystectomy with ileoconduit for invasive bladder cancer.

1. You begin your assessment and look at the transparent urostomy pouch covering the ileoconduit. The stomal opening is red and is draining urine with mucus. Is this normal?

2. The patient asks you to explain the difference between an ileoconduit and an ileostomy. How should you explain this to her?

3. A.T. is learning how to change her appliance. She tells you the stoma feels wet and it has no feeling when she touches it. Educate A.T. about the stoma.

4. What additional topics need to be addressed when doing ileoconduit teaching?

5. A.T. is quiet and sullen the third postoperative day. You ask her if something is wrong, and she confides she is concerned about whether her husband will find her attractive after he sees her "rosebud." What is the underlying problem?

CASE STUDY PROGRESS

You ask A.T. if she would love her husband or children any less if they had a physical problem that required surgical repair. She quickly tells you, "No, of course not." You suggest that her family will likely respond the same way to her surgery. You suggest that someone from the ostomate program come and talk to her.

6. What is the ostomate program?

7. A.T is well enough to begin self-care but asks you if you will change her pouch because she doesn't "want to look at it." Is there anyone on the hospital staff who could help teach A.T. ostomy self-care and offer more support?

8. A.T.'s urine looks cloudy, and another nurse suggests that you send a specimen from her pouch to the lab for analysis. Her urine does not smell foul, and she has no fever or flank pain. Should you follow through on this suggestion? Why or why not?

9. What are the signs and symptoms (S/S) of a urinary tract infection (UTI) in a patient with an ileoconduit?

10. You walk into the room and notice that A.T.'s pouch has sprung a urine leak and she has placed a washcloth over the pouch to absorb the urine. She asks you for tape to attach the washcloth to the bag. How should you respond to her request?

CASE STUDY PROGRESS

A.T. eventually masters the pouch application and is discharged home. She returns to the urology clinic in 6 months for a follow-up (F/U) visit. She has lost 24 pounds and is seen with a smaller stoma surrounded by a half-inch ring of wartlike skin. The nurse explains to A.T. that her stoma has shrunk and the bag no longer fits properly; alkaline urine washing over unprotected skin from too large an appliance opening causes a skin reaction that can either appear smooth or wartlike. The wartlike skin buildup is referred to as hyperkeratotic, hyperplastic, epitheliomatous hyperplasia, metaplasia, or acanthosis.

11. What can be done once a hyperkeratotic lesion forms around a stoma?

12. What is the proper size for an appliance for an ileoconduit?

CASE STUDY PROGRESS

A.T. mastered her ileoconduit and became a popular ostomate.

Case Study **55**

Name _____ Class/Group _____ Date _____
Group Members _____
INSTRUCTIONS All questions apply to this case study. Your responses should be brief and to the point. When asked to provide several answers, list them in order of priority or significance. Do not assume information that is not provided. Please print or write clearly. If your response is not legible, it will be marked as ? and you will need to rewrite it.

Scenario

S.M. is a 68-year-old man who is being seen at your clinic for routine health maintenance and health promotion. He reports that he has been feeling well and has no specific complaints except for some trouble "emptying my bladder." He had a CBC and complete metabolic panel (CMP) completed 1 week before his visit, and the results are as follows: Na 140 mmol/L, K 4.2 mmol/L, Cl 100 mmol/L, HCO_3 26 mmol/L, BUN 22 mg/dl, creatinine 0.8 mg/dl, glucose 94 mg/dl, RBC 5.2 million/cmm, WBC 7400 thou/cmm, Hgb 15.2 g/dl, Hct 46%, platelets 348 thou/cmm. Prostate-specific antigen (PSA) was 0.23 ng/ml, and urinalysis (UA) was within normal limits (WNL). Vital signs (VS) at this visit are 148/88, 82, 16, 96.9°F.

1. What can you tell S.M. about his lab work?

CASE STUDY PROGRESS

While obtaining your nursing history, you record no family history of cancer or other genitourinary (GU) problems. S.M. reports frequency, urgency, nocturia ×4; he has a weak stream and has to sit to void. These symptoms have been progressive over the past 6 months. He reports he was diagnosed with a large prostate a number of years ago.

2. S.M. is curious why his benign prostatic hyperplasia (BPH) would affect his urination. He is concerned he has prostate cancer. What would you teach him?

3. The primary care provider (PCP) asked for a postvoiding residual (PVR) urine test. You document that S.M. voided 60 ml and his PVR is 110 ml. What is the significance of his PVR?

4. You report the PVR to the PCP. Commonly ordered medications to treat BPH are alpha-blockers like doxazosin, terazosin, and tamsulosin (Flomax). What is the purpose of these medications?

5. The PCP ordered tamsulosin 0.4 mg/day PO. You enter S.M.'s room to teach him about this medication. What points should you include?

6. S.M. asks, "What is retrograde ejaculation?" Explain this concept.

7. "Will this condition affect my relationship with my wife?" What should you tell him?

8. What would you expect S.M. to report if the medication was successful?

CASE STUDY PROGRESS

S.M. returns in 8 months to report his symptoms are worse than ever. He has tried several different medications, but medication management failed, and he is told surgical intervention is necessary.

9. What surgical options are available to S.M.?

CASE STUDY PROGRESS

S.M. elected to undergo a Gyrus transurethral resection of the prostate (TURP). He did well postoperatively and was discharged to home.

Case Study **56**

Scenario

K.B. is a 32-year-old woman being admitted to the medical floor for complaints of (C/O) fatigue and
dehydration. While taking her history, you discover that she has diabetes mellitus (DM) and has been
insulin dependent since the age of 8. She has undergone hemodialysis (HD) for the past 3 years. Your
initial assessment of K.B. reveals a pale, thin, slightly drowsy woman. Her admitting chemistries are
Na 145 mmol/L, K 6.0 mmol/L, Cl 93 mmol/L, HCO_3 27 mmol/L, BUN 48 mg/dl, creatinine 5.0 mg/dl,
glucose 238 mg/dl. Her skin is warm and dry to touch with poor skin turgor, and her mucous membranes are dry. Her vital signs (VS) are 140/88, 116, 18, 99.9°F. She tells you she has been nauseated
for 2 days so she has not been eating or drinking. She reports severe diarrhea. Serum calcium (Ca),
phosphate (PO_4), and magnesium (Mg) have been drawn but are not yet available.

1. What aspects of your assessment support her admitting diagnosis of dehydration?

2. Identify two possible causes for K.B.'s low-grade fever.

CASE STUDY PROGRESS
The rest of K.B.'s physical assessment is within normal limits (WNL). She tells you she has an arterio-
venous (AV) fistula in her left arm.

3. What is a fistula? Why does K.B. have one?

4. In assessment of an AV fistula, what physical findings would you expect during auscultation and palpation? Why?

CASE STUDY PROGRESS

Over the next 24 hours, K.B.'s nausea subsides and she is able to eat normally. While you are helping her with her AM care, she confides in you that she doesn't understand the renal diet. "I just get blood drawn every week and meet with the dialysis dietitian every month—I just eat what she tells me to eat."

5. Because K.B. is on HD, what are her special nutritional needs?

CASE STUDY PROGRESS

K.B.'s CBC yields the following results: WBC 7.6 thou/cmm, RBC 3.2 million/cmm, Hgb 8.1 g/dl, Hct 24.3%, and platelets 333 thou/cmm.

6. Are these values normal? If not, what are the abnormalities?

7. K.B.'s physician notes that she is anemic, which most likely is the cause of her increasing fatigue. Why is K.B. anemic?

8. Patients in renal failure have the potential to develop comorbid conditions. Identify five potential problems, determine how you would assess the problem, then delineate nursing interventions and patient education strategies for each.

1. Problem:
   Assessment:

   Intervention(s):

   Patient education:

2. Problem:
   Assessment:

   Intervention(s):

   Patient education:

3. Problem:
   Assessment:

   Intervention(s):

   Patient education:

4. **Problem:**
   Assessment:

   Intervention(s):

   Patient education:

5. **Problem:**

   Assessment

   Intervention(s)

   Patient education:

6. **Problem:**
   Assessment:

   Intervention(s):

   Patient education:

7. **Problem:**
   Assessment:

   Intervention(s):

   Patient education:

CASE STUDY PROGRESS

The following day K.B. is discharged feeling much better and with a good understanding of her dietary restrictions. Her iron stores have been evaluated and found to be low. Her physician has instructed her to resume her preadmission medications, except for the addition of ferrous sulfate elixir 5 ml PO tid with meals and erythropoietin-stimulating protein (ESP) to be given 3 times a week with dialysis.

9. What information would you give K.B. about her new medications?

Case Study **57**

Name _____ **Class/Group** _____ **Date** _____
Group Members _____
INSTRUCTIONS All questions apply to this case study. Your responses should be brief and to the point. When asked to provide several answers, list them in order of priority or significance. Do not assume information that is not provided. Please print or write clearly. If your response is not legible, it will be marked as ? and you will need to rewrite it.

Scenario

A.B. is a 55-year-old man who was referred to the urology clinic by his primary care provider (PCP) for an elevated prostate-specific antigen (PSA). He reports that he has been feeling well and has no specific complaints. He had a CBC, basic metabolic panel (BMP), urinalysis (UA), lipid profile, and screening PSA completed the week before when he was seen by his PCP. His CBC, lipid profile, UA, and blood chemistries are all within normal limits (WNL); his prostate was not tender on exam, but his PSA is slightly elevated at 4.92 ng/ml.

1. A.B. wonders if he has prostate cancer. What can you tell A.B. about his PSA?

2. A.B. is scheduled for a prostate biopsy. He wonders what he needs to do to prepare for this test. Explain a prostate biopsy procedure and how to prepare for the procedure.

CASE STUDY PROGRESS

A.B.'s prostate biopsy is positive for cancer. He has discussed his diagnosis with the urologist. He is now thinking about his treatment options and asks you to answer some questions. He was told about his Gleason grade but is not sure what this is.

3. What is a Gleason grade?

4. The urologist discusses possible treatment options with A.B. Identify three treatment options for prostate cancer.

CASE STUDY PROGRESS

A.B. has decided to have his prostate removed. He is planning on having surgery in 2 weeks but is concerned about the possible consequences of surgery.

5. Identify the *major* immediate postoperative concern for A.B.

6. Identify the two main long-term consequences of prostatectomy.

7. The urologist you work for has asked you to give A.B. preoperative instructions. What should you tell him?

CASE STUDY PROGRESS

A.B. returns S/P (status post) radical prostatectomy. Initial postoperative orders include:

1. Vital signs (VS) per hospital protocol.
2. Inspect, reinforce, and change dressing according to hospital protocol.
3. NPO until after first bowel movement (BM) or passing flatus.
4. Notify physician if patient has urinary output less than 30 ml/hr, absent bowel sounds (BS), or shortness of breath (SOB).
5. Up ad lib.
6. Provide overhead irrigation as needed to maintain patent Foley catheter.
7. If Foley clots, change Foley catheter.
8. Sequential compression devices (SCDs) per hospital protocol.
9. Hemoglobin (Hgb) and hematocrit (Hct) (H/H) with PT/INR q6h × 24 hr.
10. RN to change dressing and observe epidural insertion site.
11. A.B. will return from surgery with a drain. If it has not already been done, attach a Jackson-Pratt (JP) drain to provide suction.

8. Review the list of postoperative orders. Place a star next to incorrect orders and correct them.

9. A.B. returns for his 6-month follow-up (F/U) visit. He reports he can get an erection but has difficulty maintaining an erection for sexual relations. You discuss alternative erectile aids. What options should you address?

Case Study **58**

Scenario

It is a hot summer day, and you are an RN in the emergency department (ED). S.R., an 18-year-old woman, comes to the ED with severe left flank and abdominal pain and nausea and vomiting (N/V). S.R. looks very tired, her skin is warm to touch, and she is perspiring. She paces about the room doubled-over and is clutching her abdomen. S.R. tells you that the pain started early this morning and has been pretty steady for the past 6 hours. She gives a history of working outside as a landscaper and takes little time for water breaks. Her past medical history (PMH) includes 3 kidney stone attacks, all during late summer. Exam findings are that her abdomen is soft and without tenderness, but her left flank is extremely tender to touch, palpation, and percussion. You place S.R. in one of the examination rooms and take the following vital signs (VS): 188/98, 90, 20, 99°F. Urinalysis (UA) shows RBC of 50 to 100 on voided specimen, WBC 0.

1. It is common for drug seekers to seek medical care with blood in their urine. What should you do to ensure the UA is correct?

2. The physician orders an IV pyelogram (IVP). What questions do you need to ask S.R. before the test is conducted? What do you need to check in her blood before her having an IVP?

3. S.R. states she had an allergic reaction during her last IVP and was instructed "don't let anyone give you dye for any testing." The physician cancels the IVP; what alternative test should be conducted?

CASE STUDY PROGRESS

The noncontrast CT scan shows a left 2-mm ureteral vesicle junction (UVJ) stone.

4. What are the two most common types of stones?

5. What is the most likely cause of S.R.'s stone?

6. Identify two methods of treating a patient with an UVJ stone.

CASE STUDY PROGRESS

S.R. was discharged with instructions to strain all urine and return if she experienced pain unrelieved by the pain medication or increased N/V.

7. What specific instructions will you give S.R. about her urine, fluid intake, medications, and activity?

CASE STUDY PROGRESS

S.R. returns to the ED in 6 hours with complaints of (C/O) pain unrelieved by the pain medication and increased blood in her urine. She is being held in the ED until she can be transported to surgery.

8. What is the care plan for S.R.?

CASE STUDY PROGRESS

A 2-mm calculus was removed by basket extraction. Pathologic examination reported the stone to be calcium oxalate.

9. If S.R. continues to form stones, what recommendations would an MD make for this patient?

10. Because S.R.'s stone has been reported as calcium oxalate, what type of diet would be recommended?

Case Study **59**

Name _____ Class/Group _____ Date _____

Group Members _____

INSTRUCTIONS All questions apply to this case study. Your responses should be brief and to the point. When asked to provide several answers, list them in order of priority or significance. Do not assume information that is not provided. Please print or write clearly. If your response is not legible, it will be marked as ? and you will need to rewrite it.

Scenario

F.F., a 58-year-old man with type 2 diabetes mellitus (DM) (formerly known as non–insulin-dependent DM), comes to the emergency department (ED) with severe right flank and abdominal pain and nausea and vomiting (N/V). The abdomen is soft and without tenderness. The right flank is extremely tender to touch and palpation. Vital signs (VS) are 142/80, 88, 20, 99.0°F. Urinalysis (UA) shows hematuria. An IV of 0.9 normal saline (NS) is started and set to infuse at 125 ml/hr. An IV pyelogram (IVP) confirms the diagnosis of a staghorn-type stone in the right renal pelvis. The right kidney looks enlarged. F.F. states that he did not sleep well last night and has not eaten much today. He is obviously fatigued. His laboratory results are Na 144 mmol/L, K 4.0 mmol/L, Cl 101 mmol/L, CO_2 26 mmol/L, BUN 30 mg/dl, creatinine 3.6 mg/dl, glucose 260 mg/dl, uric acid 5.0 mg/dl, Ca 9.0 units/L, phosphorus 2.6 mg/dl, total protein 7.8 g/dl, albumin 4.0 g/dl, total bilirubin 0.3 mg/dl, direct bilirubin 0.1 mg/dl, cholesterol 200 mg/dl, alkaline phosphatase 61 units/L, lactate dehydrogenase (LDH) total 100 units/L, aspartate transaminase (AST) 13 units/L, alanine transaminase (ALT) 13 units/L, gamma-glutamyl transferase (GGT) 40 units/L, amylase 98 units/L.

✷ **1.** F.F.'s pain is treated with IV morphine. It is late afternoon before he is admitted to your unit, and he is scheduled for lithotripsy in the morning. What specific priorities do you identify for F.F.?

2. The physician has prescribed gentamicin 80 mg IV piggyback (IVPB) q8h. You question the physician about giving this large of a dose of gentamicin to F.F. You are met with angry and belittling statements. Articulate your reasons for questioning this specific order for F.F.

3. How should you handle the situation with the physician to protect the patient and promote a collegial relationship?

4. A staghorn stone can cause chronic infection and renal pelvis obstruction that may result in the need for nephrectomy. How can this problem affect his long-term kidney function?

5. Analyze the relationship between creatinine and glomerular filtration rate (GFR) and prediction of kidney function.

6. Later, as you walk past his bed, you notice F.F. crawling off the end of the bed. What are you going to do?

CASE STUDY PROGRESS

F.F. is going to be admitted. You call the unit nurse to give the report. You tell her he's been up all night with pain that has just been relieved by IV morphine. You don't know whether he's going to have lithotripsy or surgery.

7. You tell F.F. he is going to be admitted and will probably need surgery for his kidney stone. He looks at you, panicked, and says, "I can't do that. I don't have any insurance. This is costing me a wad already." How are you going to respond?

✳ **Note:** *The National Kidney Disease Education Program, the Kidney Disease Outcomes Quality Initiative (KDOQI) of the National Kidney Foundation, and the Seventh Report of the Joint National Committee on Prevention, Detection, Evaluation, and Treatment of High Blood Pressure (JNC 7) all recommend use of the Modification of Diet in Renal Disease (MDRD) equation to estimate GFR in adults. A GFR calculator is available at http://www.nkdep.nih.gov or call 866-4-KIDNEY.*

Case Study **60**

Scenario

N.H., an 89-year-old widow, recently experienced a left-sided cerebrovascular accident (CVA). She has right-sided weakness and expressive aphasia with minimal swallowing difficulty. N.H. has a past medical history (PMH) of left-sided CVA 2½ years ago, chronic atrial flutter, and hypertension (HTN). She has a negative psychiatric history and has lived with her daughter's family in a rural town since her previous stroke. Since admission to an acute care facility 5 days ago, N.H. has gained some strength, has become oriented to person and place, and is anxious to begin her rehabilitation program. She is transferred for rehabilitation to your skilled nursing facility with the following orders: hydrochlorothiazide 25 mg/day PO, digoxin 0.125 mg/day PO, aspirin 81 mg/day PO, warfarin (Coumadin) 5 mg/day PO, acetaminophen (Tylenol) 325 mg q6h prn for pain, zolpidem 5 mg PO hs prn for sleep. Prescribed diet is mechanical soft, low sodium (Na) with ground meat. Other strategies are maintain Foley to down drain (DD) and then follow up with bladder training; facilitate referrals for speech, occupational, and physical therapy (OT, PT) to evaluate and treat swallowing, communication, and functional abilities.

1. What lab orders would you anticipate as a result of this specific list of orders? With each response, describe your rationale.

2. At the interdisciplinary care conferences, you report that bladder training is progressing and recommend removing the catheter if N.H.'s mobility and communication abilities have progressed sufficiently. The group and N.H. agree that she is ready for the Foley catheter to be removed. Identify three problems that N.H. is at risk for developing following catheter removal. Describe specific interventions for each problem.

❋ 3. Two days after the Foley is removed, you observe that N.H.'s urine is cloudy, is concentrated, and has a strong odor. What are your immediate actions?

4. N.H. is started on sulfamethoxazole 800 mg/trimethoprim 160 mg (Bactrim DS) 1 tab PO bid × 10 days. However, 2 days later N.H. is in the bathroom, and she is very upset. There is blood on the toilet, and the water is bright red with blood. You help the CNA clean N.H. and help her into bed. Describe your assessment steps. What complications do you anticipate?

5. You complete your assessment and report your findings to the physician. You obtain an order for a straight catheterized urine specimen for C&S. Identify at least two potential causes for N.H.'s hematuria.

6. N.H.'s urinary tract infection (UTI) is responding to antibiotics, and you want to prepare her and her daughter for eventual discharge. What specific issues must be considered in the teaching and discharge planning to prevent a recurrence of infection?

7. You talk with N.H.'s daughter about her understanding of caregiving responsibilities for her mother. What kind of questions do you ask to assess whether she is capable of taking on this additional burden?

chapter 6

Neurologic Disorders

Case Study 61

Name _____ Class/Group _____ Date _____
Group Members _____

INSTRUCTIONS All questions apply to this case study. Your responses should be brief and to the point. When asked to provide several answers, list them in order of priority or significance. Do not assume information that is not provided. Please print or write clearly. If your response is not legible, it will be marked as ? and you will need to rewrite it.

Scenario

M.E. is a 62-year-old woman who has a 5-year history of progressive forgetfulness. She is no longer able to care for herself, has become increasingly depressed and paranoid, and recently started a fire in the kitchen. After extensive neurologic evaluation, M.E. is diagnosed as having Alzheimer's disease. Her husband and children have come to the Alzheimer's unit at your extended care facility for information about this disease and to discuss the possibility of placement for M.E. You reassure the family that you have experience dealing with the questions and concerns of most people in their situation.

1. How would you explain Alzheimer's disease to the family?

2. The husband asks, "How did she get Alzheimer's? We don't know anyone else who has it." How would you respond?

3. After asking the family to describe M.E.'s behavior, you determine that she is in stage 5 of Alzheimer's 7 stages. Describe common signs and symptoms (S/S) for each stage of the disease.

Stage 1

Stage 2

Stage 3

Stage 4

Stage 5

Stage 6

Stage 7

4. The daughter expresses frustration at the number of tests M.E. had to undergo and the length of time it took for someone to diagnose M.E.'s problem. What tests are likely to be performed, and how is Alzheimer's disease diagnosed?

CASE STUDY PROGRESS

M.E.'s husband states, "How are you going to take care of her? She wanders around all night long. She can't find her way to the bathroom in a house she's lived in for 43 years. She can't be trusted to be alone any more; she almost burnt the house down. We're all exhausted; there are 3 of us, and we can't keep up with her." You acknowledge how exhausted they must be from trying to keep her safe. You tell the family that there is no known treatment, but Alzheimer's units have been created to provide a structured, safe environment for each person.

5. Describe the Alzheimer's-related nursing interventions R/T (related to) each of the following nursing care problems: self-care deficits, sleep pattern disturbance, impaired verbal communication, impaired cognitive function, risk for injury, and agitation.

6. M.E.'s son asks what different medications might be prescribed for M.E. How would you describe the purpose of antiseizure, cognitive, antipsychotic, anticonvulsant, antidepressant, sedative, antianxiety, and other medications for a patient like M.E.?

CASE STUDY PROGRESS

You try to comfort the family by telling them that the problems they are experiencing are common. You explain that family support is a major focus of your program.

7. List four ways that M.E.'s family might receive the support they need.

Case Study **62**

Scenario

C.B. is a 58-year-old man with Guillain-Barré syndrome (GBS). He was transferred to a skilled nursing facility that cares for patients requiring mechanical ventilation 2 days ago. C.B. is a single, self-supporting man from a small town. He came to see his family physician in early January with symptoms of fatigue, myalgia, fever, and chills, which were accompanied by a hacking cough. He was diagnosed with viral influenza. Three weeks later he developed bilateral weakness, numbness, and tingling of his lower extremities, which rapidly progressed into his upper body. He was brought to the emergency department (ED) after his brother recognized the seriousness of his condition. Shortly after arrival he became totally paralyzed and required endotracheal intubation and mechanical ventilation. He was then admitted to the neurology critical care unit, where he spent 1 month. He underwent a tracheotomy before being transferred to a medical floor, where he spent several weeks. He was treated for pneumonia while hospitalized on the medical floor. His pneumonia resolved before transfer to a skilled care facility for further rehabilitation and continued ventilatory support.

1. What is the etiology of GBS?

2. What type of individual is likely to be diagnosed with GBS?

3. What are the clinical manifestations of GBS?

4. Is C.B.'s case typical?

5. How is GBS diagnosed?

6. Why does life-threatening respiratory dysfunction occur?

7. How would C.B.'s nutritional needs be maintained?

8. What interventions can you implement to decrease C.B.'s fear and anxiety?

9. What is the medical management for GBS?

Case Study **63**

Name _____ Class/Group _____ Date _____
Group Members _____

INSTRUCTIONS All questions apply to this case study. Your responses should be brief and to the point. When asked to provide several answers, list them in order of priority or significance. Do not assume information that is not provided. Please print or write clearly. If your response is not legible, it will be marked as ? and you will need to rewrite it.

Scenario

L.C. is a 78-year-old white man with a 4-year history of Parkinson's disease (PD). He is a retired engineer, is married, and lives with his wife in a small farming community. He has 4 adult children who live close by. He is taking carbidopa-levodopa, pergolide, and amantadine. L.C. reports that overall he is doing "about the same" as he was at his last clinic visit 6 months ago. He reports that his tremor is about the same, his gait is perhaps a little more unsteady, and his fatigue is slightly more noticeable. L.C. is also concerned about increased drooling. The patient and his wife report that he is taking carbidopa-levodopa 25/100 mg (Sinemet), 1 tablet an hour before breakfast and 1 tablet 2 hours after lunch, and carbidopa-levodopa 50/200 mg (Sinemet CR), 1 tablet at bedtime. On the previous visit they were encouraged to try taking the carbidopa-levodopa (Sinemet) more times throughout the day, but they report that he became very somnolent with that dosing regimen. He also reports that his dyskinetic movements appear to be worse just after taking his carbidopa-levodopa.

1. What is parkinsonism?

2. What is PD?

3. What are the clinical manifestations of PD? Place a star next to the symptoms L.C. has mentioned.

4. L.C.'s wife asks you, "How do the doctors know L.C. has Parkinson's disease? They never did a lot of tests on him." How is the diagnosis of PD made?

5. L.C.'s wife comments "I don't even know which one of his medicines he takes for his Parkinson's." What medications are used for PD?

6. L.C. asks, "If I don't have enough dopamine, then why don't they give me a dopamine pill?" Why can't oral DA be given as replacement therapy?

7. Levodopa is always given in combination with carbidopa. Why?

8. What is the current recommended nutritional management for PD?

9. L.C.'s wife is getting their belongings together to leave when she asks, "They can do surgery for everything else. Why can't they do surgery to fix Parkinson's?" What types of surgical treatments are available for patients with PD?

10. What are three interventions that should be implemented in caring for L.C.?

11. You are a case manager. Identify six things that you would assess to determine if L.C. could be cared for in his home.

Case Study **64**

Name _____ Class/Group_____ Date _____

Group Members _____

INSTRUCTIONS All questions apply to this case study. Your responses should be brief and to the point. When asked to provide several answers, list them in order of priority or significance. Do not assume information that is not provided. Please print or write clearly. If your response is not legible, it will be marked as ? and you will need to rewrite it.

Scenario

It is early morning and N.T., a 79-year-old woman, is getting out of bed. She has a mild headache over the right temple, is fatigued, and feels slightly weak. She calls for her husband to let him know she will be going back to bed for a while. When her husband comes in to check on her, he finds that she is having trouble saying words and has a slight left-sided facial droop. When he helps her up from the bedside, he notices weakness in her left hand and convinces her to go to the local emergency department (ED). Her first CT scan was negative for cerebrovascular accident (CVA); however, the second CT scan (18 hours later) reveals a small CVA in the right hemisphere. She is still experiencing expressive aphasia, left facial droop, left-sided hemiparesis, and what is presumed to be symptoms of mild dysphagia. Her past medical history (PMH) includes paroxysmal atrial fibrillation (PAF), hypertension (HTN), hyperlipidemia, and a remote history (Hx) of deep vein thrombosis (DVT). A recent cardiac stress test was normal, and her blood pressure (BP) has been well controlled. She admits to being under recent stress with the death of her husband's adult son. She is hospitalized for 4 days and discharged with orders for outpatient rehabilitation for speech and physical therapy (PT). Medications she took before the CVA were flecainide (Tambocor), hormone replacement therapy (HRT), amlodipine (Norvasc), aspirin, simvastatin (Zocor), and trandolapril (Mavik). She is discharged on flecainide, amlodipine, clopidogrel (Plavix), aspirin, simvastatin, and trandolapril.

1. What other information would be necessary for evaluating the *cause* for the CVA?

2. If her deficits are temporary, how long might it take before they are completely reversed?

3. Why was N.T. placed on clopidogrel post–CVA?

4. Why was the initial CT scan negative for stroke?

5. N.T. is not on HRT post-CVA. Why would this medication be discontinued?

6. Is there any benefit from continuing simvastatin after her CVA?

7. Is there treatment that can be initiated in the ED to stop a CVA from progressing?

8. Your co-worker states, "I always heard that PAF is a precursor to stroke." Is this statement true or false?

9. Which of the following is not a symptom of CVA?
1. Headache
2. Lethargy
3. Lumbar pain
4. Blurred vision

10. As you walk into the nurses' station, the charge nurse is talking to N.T.'s physician, who ordered a modified barium swallow study and referral for speech-language pathologist (SLP), occupational therapist (OT), and registered dietitian (RD). Give the rationale for these orders.

11. What lab test may be abnormal during CVA?

12. N.T.'s BP should be well controlled. What BP level should be considered normal for her, based on the Seventh Report of the Joint National Committee on Prevention, Detection, Evaluation, and Treatment of High Blood Pressure (JNC 7)?

Case Study **66**

Name _____ Class/Group _____ Date _____
Group Members _____
INSTRUCTIONS All questions apply to this case study. Your responses should be brief and to the point. When asked
to provide several answers, list them in order of priority or significance. Do not assume information that is not provided.
Please print or write clearly. If your response is not legible, it will be marked as ? and you will need to rewrite it.

Scenario

J.B. is a 58-year-old retired postal worker who has been on your floor for several days receiving plasmapheresis every other day for myasthenia gravis (MG). Before this admission, he had been relatively healthy. His medical history includes hypertension (HTN) controlled with metoprolol and glaucoma treated with timolol (ophthalmic preparation). About a year ago, J.B. started experiencing difficulty chewing and swallowing, diplopia, and slurring of speech, at which time he was placed on pyridostigmine (Mestinon). Recently J.B. was diagnosed with a sinus infection and treated with ciprofloxacin. On admission, J.B. was unable to bear any weight or take fluids through a straw. There have been periods of exacerbation and remission since admission.

1. J.B.'s wife asks you, "What may have caused my husband to get worse?" What explanation should you give her?

2. You are visiting with J.B.'s wife, who tells you she doesn't have a lot of information about MG and she would like to know more about it so that she will feel more comfortable talking to her husband. What should you tell her?

3. J.B.'s wife asks you to explain what to expect in terms of S/S as her husband's illness progresses. What should you tell her?

4. J.B.'s wife asks how this disease is diagnosed. "How do they know that my husband has MG?" What should you tell her?

5. J.B.'s wife asks, "What are some options for treatment of MG?" How should you explain the different treatments?

6. List four factors that could predispose J.B. to an exacerbation of his illness.

7. J.B.'s wife asks what the physicians and nurses watch for while her husband is in the hospital. How should you explain these activities?

8. J.B.'s wife wants to know when he will be able to go home. How should you respond?

9. J.B.'s wife asks you what information she will need before taking her husband home. How should you explain this to her?

10. J.B.'s wife asks you, "What is the difference between cholinergic crisis and myasthenic crisis?" What explanation should you give her?

11. What supportive measures can you suggest to J.B.'s wife that she can undertake or arrange on behalf of her husband?

For further information contact:

American Autoimmune Related Diseases Association: *http://www.aarda.org*; (810) 776-3900, (800) 598-4668

Myasthenia Gravis Foundation of America: *http://www.myasthenia.org*; (800) 541-5454

National Institute of Neurological Disorders and Stroke: *http://www.ninds.nih.gov*

National Women's Health Information Center: *http://www.WomensHealth.gov*; (800) 994-9662

Case Study **67**

Name _____ Class/Group _____ Date _____
Group Members _____
INSTRUCTIONS All questions apply to this case study. Your responses should be brief and to the point. When asked to provide several answers, list them in order of priority or significance. Do not assume information that is not provided. Please print or write clearly. If your response is not legible, it will be marked as ? and you will need to rewrite it.

Scenario

You have been asked to see D.V. in the neurology clinic. D.V. has been referred by his internist, who thinks his patient is having symptoms of multiple sclerosis (MS). D.V. is a 25-year-old man who has experienced increasing urinary frequency and urgency over the past 2 months. Because his female partner was treated for a sexually transmitted disease (STD), D.V. also underwent treatment, but the symptoms did not resolve. D.V. has also recently had 2 brief episodes of eye "fuzziness" associated with diplopia and brightness. He has noticed ascending numbness and weakness of the right arm with inability to hold objects over the past few days. Now he reports rapid progression of weakness in his legs.

1. MS is an inflammatory disorder of the nervous system causing scattered, patchy demyelinization of the central nervous system (CNS). What does myelin do? What is demyelinization?

2. MS is characterized by remissions and exacerbations. What happens to the myelin during each of these phases?

3. Isn't D.V. too young to get MS? What is the etiology?

4. What assessment data caused the physician to suspect a possible diagnosis of MS?

✻ **Note:** *Diagnostic tests are often done to rule out (R/O) other disorders with similar symptoms. A diagnosis will be made when other disorders have been R/O; when the patient has 2 or more exacerbations; when there is slow, steady progression; and when the patient has 2 or more areas of demyelinization or plaque formation.*

5. What are four common diagnostic tests you can begin to teach D.V. about?

6. D.V. asks you, "If this turns out to be MS, what is the treatment?"

7. As part of your teaching plan, you want D.V. to be aware of situations or factors that are known to exacerbate symptoms. List four.

CASE STUDY PROGRESS

D.V. confides in you that he has been depressed since his parents' divorce and the onset of these symptoms. He tells you that he knows his girlfriend hasn't been faithful, but he's afraid of living alone. He's afraid if he tells her about his MS diagnosis, she'll leave him.

8. What are you going to do with this information?

9. In view of his personal history and current diagnosis, what two critical psychosocial issues are you going to monitor in his follow-up (F/U) visits?

10. List several resources available in the community that D.V. may find helpful.

CASE STUDY PROGRESS

D.V. takes advantage of his time with the psychiatric nurse specialist, joins a local MS support group, and tells his girlfriend to move out. He later marries a woman from the support group.

For additional information, contact:

Multiple Sclerosis Association of America: (800) 532-7667

National Multiple Sclerosis Society: *http://www.nationalmssociety.org;* (800) 344-4867

Case Study **68**

Name _____ Class/Group _____ Date _____
Group Members _____
INSTRUCTIONS All questions apply to this case study. Your responses should be brief and to the point. When asked
to provide several answers, list them in order of priority or significance. Do not assume information that is not provided.
Please print or write clearly. If your response is not legible, it will be marked as ? and you will need to rewrite it.

Scenario

J.G. is a 34-year-old P1G1 (para 1, gravida 1) woman who underwent an emergency cesarean delivery
after a prolonged labor, during which she exhibited a sudden change in neurologic functioning and
started seizing. Since that time, she has experienced 3 tonic-clonic (grand mal) seizures. She was diagnosed as having a basal ganglion hematoma with infarct and was started on phenytoin. Postdelivery,
J.G. demonstrated dyskinesia, resulting in frequent falls during ambulation. Once the seizure disorder
appeared to be under control, she was transferred to a rehabilitation facility for evaluation and 2 weeks
of intensive physical therapy (PT). She is now home, where she is doing well but still has occasional
falls, and is receiving PT 3 times a week in her home. She remains on phenytoin and has had no seizures
since her release from the rehabilitation facility. As case manager (CM) for J.G.'s health maintenance
organization (HMO), you make a home visit with her and her family for evaluation of long-term, follow-
up (F/U) care.

1. A seizure is not a disease in itself but a symptom of a disease. What is the term for
   chronically recurring seizures?

2. Does J.G. have epilepsy?

3. The three main phases of a seizure are the preictal, ictal, and postictal. Differentiate among
   the three phases, and list clinical symptoms you might observe when a patient is having a
   seizure.

4. What is the pathophysiology of a seizure?

5. J.G. had tonic–clonic, or grand mal, seizures. Describe this type of seizure. List five other types of seizures.

6. Some patients know they are about to have a seizure. What is this preseizure warning called, and what form does it take?

7. Besides the brain injury, what are some other possible conditions that could be contributing to J.G.'s lowered seizure threshold?

8. List five different classifications of antiepileptic drugs (AEDs) or antiseizure medications.

9. You are the CM making a home visit. While you are there, J.G.'s husband asks you what he should do if she has a seizure at home. What do you tell him?

10. Her husband states that he is afraid for J.G. to take care of the baby. What would you say to him?

11. J.G.'s husband tells you that his wife is not good at remembering to take medication. What are some strategies that you should review with J.G. and her husband to increase the likelihood of compliance?

12. J.G. asks, "If I get my blood level under control, will it stay at the same level as long as I take my medicine?" How would you answer her question?

13. J.G.'s husband asks whether the drugs could harm his wife in any way. What general information would you give them about anticonvulsants?

14. J.G.'s husband says, "I was watching a TV show set in a hospital last night, and they showed this guy who just kept on having a seizure. That doctor had to give him lots of medicine before he came out of it." How would you explain status epilepticus, and why is it a medical emergency?

Bonus Problem

Look up the MedicAlert website, and plan a 10-minute presentation for patients, consumers, and families on the importance of people with seizure disorders wearing standardized identification. Include instructions on cost, benefits, and how to obtain MedicAlert identification.

For additional information contact:
MedicAlert Foundation International: *http://www.medicalert.org*; (888) 633-4298
Other helpful organizations for seizure and epilepsy include:
American Epilepsy Society: *http://www.aesnet.org*; (860) 586-7505
Epilepsy Foundation: *http://www.epilepsyfoundation.org*; (800) 332-1000

Case Study **69**

Name _____ Class/Group _____ Date _____
Group Members _____
INSTRUCTIONS All questions apply to this case study. Your responses should be brief and to the point. When asked to provide several answers, list them in order of priority or significance. Do not assume information that is not provided. Please print or write clearly. If your response is not legible, it will be marked as ? and you will need to rewrite it.

Scenario

F.N. is a 57-year-old housewife, happily married with grown children and 2 new grandchildren. F.N. made an appointment with her optometrist to explore a progressive OS (left eye) visual loss over a 9-month period. Her eye exam was essentially normal, and the optometrist referred her to a neurologist. After work-up, a 2.5-cm brain mass was found, and surgery was scheduled. Her only past medical history (PMH) is hypertension (HTN), for which she takes long-acting metoprolol (Toprol XL) 100 mg/day. Her past surgical history (PSH) includes tonsillectomy and adenoidectomy (T&A) as a child, cholecystectomy, and a total abdominal hysterectomy (TAH) at age 42. She also takes a conjugated estrogen (Premarin) 0.625 mg/day.

1. Name one test that can be done to evaluate for brain tumor.

✳ **Note:** *There is no standardized, universally accepted system of classifying brain tumors. They can be classified on a histologic basis, intraaxial versus extraaxial, or malignant versus benign.*

2. Using the term *benign* when discussing brain tumors is somewhat misleading. Why?

3. Onset of neurologic symptoms is usually insidious, and patients exhibit symptoms in relation to the area of the brain where the tumor is located. List six general symptoms associated with many brain tumors.

4. Corticosteroids, such as dexamethasone (Decadron), prednisone (Deltasone), or methylprednisolone (Solu-Medrol), are commonly prescribed when a tumor is diagnosed and the presence of increase intracranial pressure (ICP) is demonstrated. The drugs are administered preoperatively and postoperatively and in conjunction with radiation and chemotherapy. Why is dexamethasone prescribed, and why should it not be abruptly stopped?

5. Other common supportive medications include anticonvulsants, diuretics (including osmotic diuretics), H$_2$ blockers, analgesics, antiemetics, and antidepressants. Indicate why each is used.

6. Once the diagnosis is made, the patient and family must be involved in the plan for treatment. Treatment depends on the type, grade, and location of the tumor and can include surgery, radiation, chemotherapy, or any combination of these. The patient also has the right to refuse treatment. Identify four other factors the medical team, patient, and family would consider in devising a treatment plan.

7. Describe common responses to a diagnosis of a brain tumor.

8. F.N. draws up a living will and health care power of attorney after she hears the diagnosis. She also sits down with her family and makes her wishes known. Why is this important for F.N. in particular and for everyone in general?

9. You enter F.N.'s room to take vital signs (VS), and she says, "What if I come out of surgery and I'm different? Or what if I die? My grandbabies will never know me." You hear the concern in her voice and want to provide realistic reassurance about expected outcomes. Suggest several ways that F.N. can communicate with her loved ones in the event that her surgery is unsuccessful.

10. F.N. has the surgery and is admitted to ICU postoperatively. She does very well and remains neurologically intact (neurologic checks every hour). Her blood pressure (BP) is slightly elevated (147/68 mm Hg); the rest of her VS are normal; she has two peripheral IVs, TED (thromboembolic deterrent) hose, oxygen (O_2) at 4 L by nasal cannula (NC), and a Foley. Postoperatively, F.N.'s potassium (K) level drops to 2.7 mmol/L, and glucose is 202 mg/dl. Describe possible reasons why these 2 laboratory values are abnormal, and identify what treatment will be ordered to correct each.

CASE STUDY PROGRESS

F.N. did suffer mild neurologic damage as a result of the surgery. She was discharged to a rehabilitation facility and eventually recovered most of her lost function. She continues to enjoy an active life and has become involved in helping others face similar experiences.

For additional information contact:

American Brain Tumor Association: *http://hope.abta.org;* (800) 886-2282

American Cancer Society: *http://www.cancer.org;* (800) ACS-2345

Cancer Information Service: *http://cis.nci.nih.gov;* (800) 4-CANCER

National Brain Tumor Foundation: *http://www.braintumor.org;* (800) 934-CURE

Case Study **70**

Name _____ Class/Group _____ Date _____
Group Members _____
INSTRUCTIONS All questions apply to this case study. Your responses should be brief and to the point. When asked
to provide several answers, list them in order of priority or significance. Do not assume information that is not provided.
Please print or write clearly. If your response is not legible, it will be marked as ? and you will need to rewrite it.

Scenario

T.W. is a 22-year-old man who fell 50 feet from a chairlift while skiing and landed on hard-packed
snow. He was found to have a T10-11 fracture with paraplegia. He was initially admitted to the surgical
intensive care unit (SICU) from the emergency department (ED) and placed on high-dose steroids for
24 hours. He was taken to surgery 48 hours after the accident for spinal stabilization. He spent 2
additional days in the SICU and 5 days on the neurologic unit, and now is ready to be transferred to
your rehab unit. He continues to have no movement of his lower extremities.

1. Awareness of the prehospital management of a spinal cord injury (SCI) is critical to each
   patient's ultimate neurologic outcome. What actions should the nurse take to ensure this
   goal is met?

✳ 2. On arrival to the ED, what are the main interventions done by the ED nurse?

3. T.W. receives high-dose steroid therapy in the ED; then he is placed on a continuous infusion. What effect will steroids have on T.W., and what is the usual method of steroid administration?

4. List three critical potential infections that T.W. should be monitored for throughout his hospitalization.

5. Explain the difference between spinal shock and neurogenic shock.

　✳ **Note:** *A person with an SCI at the T10-12 level should be independent in a wheelchair (W/C) and able to manage activities of daily living (ADLs), including bowel and bladder care.*

6. T.W. is taking vitamin C 1 to 2 g qid. What is the purpose of this?

CASE STUDY PROGRESS

You request a consultation with a registered dietitian (RD) because you realize that T.W. needs proteins for healing; however, too much protein can stress his kidneys. The RD will adjust his diet to ensure adequate amounts of protein, carbohydrates, calcium, thiamine, niacin, vitamins B$_6$ and D, magnesium, and zinc (see *http://www.spinalcord.org*).

7. Rehabilitation teaching includes teaching T.W. how to manage his urinary drainage system. What would this teaching include?

8. When can the bladder training program be started?

9. The large bowel musculature has its own neural center that can directly respond to distention caused by fecal material. This is what allows most SCI patients to regain bowel control. What dietary instructions are important for T.W.?

10. T.W. should also be taught bowel training techniques. What would this teaching include?

11. What medications can assist with a bowel program?

12. Describe digital stimulation.

13. T.W. asks you whether he'll ever be able to have sex again. What do you tell him, and what are some possible referrals?

CASE STUDY PROGRESS

For patients with lesions at T6 or above, there is the potential for autonomic dysreflexia (AD). Noxious stimulus below the level of injury triggers the sympathetic nervous system, causing massive release of catecholamines and producing vasoconstriction below the lesion. The patient develops severe hypertension (HTN) (as high as 240/120 mm Hg or higher), pounding headache, bradycardia, blurred vision, nausea, nasal congestion, and flushing and sweating above the level of the injury and goose bumps or pallor below the level of the injury.

14. What are potential causes of AD?

15. What are interventions related to (R/T) AD?

16. AD is a medical emergency. What could happen if it is left untreated?

❊ **17.** Consider a hierarchy of rehabilitation needs for patients such as T.W. Number the following options from highest (1) to lowest (8) priority as they apply to T.W.
____ A. Community integration
____ B. Gainful employment
____ C. Accomplishment of self-care and ADLs
____ D. Self-actualization
____ E. Stabilization of the physiologic systems and early psychologic support
____ F. Adjustment to living at home
____ G. Participation of physical therapy, occupational therapy, and social worker; use of assistive devices; bowel and bladder training
____ H. Independence

For additional information, contact:
National Spinal Cord Injury Association: *http://www.spinalcord.org*; (800) 962-9629

Case Study **71**

Scenario

Y.W. is a 23-year-old male student from Thailand studying electrical engineering at the university. He
was ejected from a moving vehicle, which was traveling 70 mph. His injuries included a severe closed
head injury with an occipital hematoma, bilateral wrist fractures, and a right pneumothorax. During
his neurologic intensive care unit (NICU) stay, Y.W. was intubated and placed on mechanical ventilation,
had a feeding tube inserted and was placed on tube feedings, had a Foley catheter to down drain
(DD), and had multiple IVs inserted. He developed pneumonia 1 month after admission.

1. Define the term *primary head injury*.

2. Define the term *secondary head injury*.

3. What is normal intracranial pressure (ICP), and why is increased ICP so clinically
important?

4. Identify at least five signs and symptoms (S/S) of increased ICP.

5. List 4 medication classifications that the ICU nurses could use to decrease or control increased ICP.

6. List 8 nursing measures that the ICU nurses could use to decrease or control increased ICP.

7. Y.W.'s medication list includes clindamycin 150 mg per feeding tube q6h, ranitidine (Zantac elixir) 150 mg per feeding tube bid, and phenytoin (Dilantin) 100 mg IV piggyback (IVPB) tid. Indicate the reasons for each.

✳ **Note:** *Do not put medications into the feeding bag with the formula because:*
- *The drug can precipitate the formula and clog the tubing.*
- *You do not know whether the patient received the entire dose of the medication.*
- *Depending on the rate of delivery, it may take hours to deliver the medication, and you may end up with several doses or multiple medications in the feeding bag.*

  Usually medication is given through the PEG tube. Disconnect the feeding, flush the tubing, deliver the medication, flush the tubing between and after each medication, then clamp the tubing or reconnect the feeding as appropriate.

8. A STAT portable chest x-ray (CXR) is ordered after each central venous catheter (CVC) is inserted. According to hospital protocol, no one is permitted to infuse anything through the catheter until the CXR has been read by the physician or radiologist. What is the purpose of the CXR, and why isn't fluid infused through the catheter until after the CXR is read?

CASE STUDY PROGRESS
Y.W. spent 2 months in acute care and is now on your rehabilitation unit. He follows commands but tends to get agitated with too much stimulation. His tracheostomy site is well healed, and the pneumonia is finally resolving. He is still receiving supplemental tube feeding and has some continued incontinence of both bowel and bladder. Y.W. has a supportive group of friends who are students at the university; several of them are also from Thailand.

9. Y.W.'s latest lab results are as follows: Na 149 mmol/L, K 4.2 mmol/L, Cl 119 mmol/L, total CO_2 21 mmol/L, BUN 12 mg/dl, creatinine 1.2 mg/dl, glucose 123 mg/dl, WBC 15.4 thou/cmm, Hgb 14.9 g/dl, Hct 36.4%, platelets 140 thou/cmm. Are any of these of concern to you, and what would you suggest to correct them?

10. Are you surprised by Y.W.'s agitated behavior? Explain.

11. Outline a general rehabilitation plan for Y.W. based on the above data.

12. Y.W.'s mother has just arrived in the United States and speaks no English. What measures can be taken to facilitate communication between medical personnel and the mother?

13. Y.W.'s mother will need a place to stay while in the United States. What can you do to facilitate the initial contact with the Thai community?

14. What special discharge planning considerations are there in this case?

Case Study **72**

Name _____ Class/Group _____ Date _____
Group Members _____

INSTRUCTIONS All questions apply to this case study. Your responses should be brief and to the point. When asked to provide several answers, list them in order of priority or significance. Do not assume information that is not provided. Please print or write clearly. If your response is not legible, it will be marked as ? and you will need to rewrite it.

Scenario

K.B. is a 21-year-old man with a past medical history (PMH) of seizure disorder controlled with carbamazepine (Tegretol). He was accidentally struck in the head by a pitched baseball while batting in a baseball game. He was unconscious momentarily, about 5 seconds, then awakened and was alert and responsive. After a few hours, K.B. returned home with complaints of a "splitting" headache, drowsiness, slight confusion, and some nausea. K.B. was taken to the local hospital emergency department (ED), where a CT scan revealed a left subdural hematoma. He has been transferred to your medical center, which has a neurosurgeon on call.

1. The ED RN gives you the above information during a phoned report. What other information do you need to prepare for this patient?

2. Because you occasionally have trouble remembering the layers of the brain and different hematomas, you look up subdural hematoma before K.B. arrives. What do you find?

3. K.B.'s subdural hematoma is considered acute because symptoms appeared within 24 to 48 hours of injury. What are the other classifications of subdural hematomas?

4. What are common signs and symptoms (S/S) of an acute subdural hematoma?

5. Why are the elderly and alcoholics at risk for chronic subdural hematomas?

6. What neurologic changes and indicators would you monitor in K.B. for increased intracranial pressure (ICP)?

7. Why is it especially important to make certain K.B. is taking his carbamazepine and has a therapeutic serum level?

8. The decision was made, in K.B.'s case, not to do a craniotomy. When would a neurosurgeon decide to treat medically versus perform surgery?

9. Why would hypotonic IV solutions such as D$_5$W be avoided in K.B.?

10. How would you position K.B. in bed to help control ICP?

11. What other interventions would be appropriate to implement in the care of K.B.?

12. K.B.'s LOC started to decrease. What information would you provide to the neurosurgeon when you call?

13. How would you support the family?

Case Study **73**

Name _____ Class/Group _____ Date _____
Group Members _____

INSTRUCTIONS All questions apply to this case study. Your responses should be brief and to the point. When asked to provide several answers, list them in order of priority or significance. Do not assume information that is not provided. Please print or write clearly. If your response is not legible, it will be marked as ? and you will need to rewrite it.

Scenario

C.J. is a 22-year-old concert pianist and is scheduled to perform tonight. Before her performance, she told a friend that she was experiencing what she called "the worst headache I've ever had." She decides that she must perform despite the pain, and she takes 2 extra-strength acetaminophens (Tylenol ES). During her performance, she stops playing, reaches up to grasp her head, then falls unconscious. When the paramedics arrive, she is intubated, an IV is started with normal saline (NS), and her ECG reveals a sinus tachycardia.

On arrival to the emergency department (ED), she has a Glasgow Coma Scale score of 3. Her husband reports a history of hypertension (HTN) and states she recently quit taking her medication because it made her feel tired. She is trying to quit smoking; she has cut down to a half pack of cigarettes per day, she drinks alcohol only socially on weekends, and she has a remote history of cocaine use. He says that she has complained of worsening, intermittent headaches for the past few weeks.

1. What is the Glasgow Coma Scale?

2. What is a subarachnoid hemorrhage (SAH)?

3. What are the causes of a SAH?

4. What are C.J.'s risk factors for SAH?

5. How is the diagnosis of SAH made?

6. How are SAHs graded?

7. What kinds of aneurysms cause SAH?

CASE STUDY PROGRESS

Once the CT scan is done on C.J., the diagnosis of SAH is made and she is transported to the ICU and closely monitored.

8. What are the main complications associated with SAH?

9. Identify the treatment given after SAH to prevent the above complications.

10. What is the recommended treatment for SAH?

11. What considerations should be made for patients with SAH?

Case Study **74**

Name _____ Class/Group _____ Date _____
Group Members _____

INSTRUCTIONS All questions apply to this case study. Your responses should be brief and to the point. When asked to provide several answers, list them in order of priority or significance. Do not assume information that is not provided. Please print or write clearly. If your response is not legible, it will be marked as ? and you will need to rewrite it.

Scenario

D.H., a 54-year-old resort owner, has had multiple chronic medical problems, including type 2 diabetes mellitus (DM) for 25 years, which has progressed to insulin-dependent DM for the past 10 years; a kidney transplant 5 years ago with no signs of rejection at last biopsy; hypertension (HTN); and remote peptic ulcer disease (PUD). His medications include insulin, immunosuppressive agents, and two anti-hypertensive drugs. He visited his local physician with complaints of (C/O) left ear, mastoid, and sinus pain. He was diagnosed with sinusitis and *Candida albicans* infection (thrush); cephalexin and nystatin were prescribed. Later that evening he developed nausea and vomiting (N/V), hematemesis, and weakness, and he was taken to the emergency department (ED). He was admitted and started on IV antibiotics, but his condition worsened throughout the night; his dyspnea increased and he developed difficulty speaking. He was flown to your tertiary referral center and was intubated en route. On arrival, D.H. had decreased level of consciousness (LOC) with periods of total unresponsiveness, weakness, and cranial nerve deficits. His diagnosis is meningitis complicated by an aspiration pneumonia and atrial fibrillation. D.H. has continued fever and leukocytosis despite aggressive antibiotic therapy.

1. Why is D.H. at particular risk for infection?

2. Describe bacterial meningitis.

3. What is the probable route of entry of bacteria into D.H.'s brain?

4. How do you think D.H. might have developed aspiration pneumonia?

5. What factors influenced the physician's decision to transport D.H. from a smaller hospital to a tertiary referral center?

6. Name four tests that could be used in the diagnosis of meningitis.

7. D.H. is taking the following medications: NPH insulin and sliding-scale regular insulin, sucralfate (Carafate), azathioprine (Imuran), imipenem and cilastatin sodium (Primaxin), methylprednisolone (Solu–Medrol), digoxin, and metronidazole (Flagyl). Indicate why he is receiving each medication.

8. The lab just called you with a glucose result of 350 mg/dl. Identify two factors that could contribute to D.H.'s elevated glucose level.

9. List seven interventions for management of D.H.'s current problems.

10. List six interventions given to prevent complications.

11. D.H.'s family is staying at a nearby motel. His adult son brings his mother to the hospital. Mrs. H. says she just wants to stay with her husband around the clock. She states, "I took care of him for 35 years now, and I'm not going to abandon him now when he needs me the most." How would you respond?

✳ **Note:** *These are stressful times for all individuals involved. Anything nurses can do to help alleviate the stress contributes to the well-being of patients and families. In these situations, you might consider asking if the family would like to talk with a spiritual counselor.*

CASE STUDY PROGRESS

D.H.'s infection destroyed his cadaver kidney. He developed multiple system organ failure (MSOF) and died 7 weeks later.

For more information contact:

Center for Disease Control and Prevention: *http://www.cdc.gov*

National Center for Infectious Diseases: *http://www.cdc.gov/ncidod*

Case Study **75**

Name _____ Class/Group _____ Date _____
Group Members _____
INSTRUCTIONS All questions apply to this case study. Your responses should be brief and to the point. When asked to provide several answers, list them in order of priority or significance. Do not assume information that is not provided. Please print or write clearly. If your response is not legible, it will be marked as ? and you will need to rewrite it.

Scenario

S.B. is a 17-year-old man who lost control of his SUV (sport utility vehicle) and struck a tree. Witnesses reported he was not restrained, and his face hit the windshield on impact. When paramedics arrived, S.B. was responsive but confused, had significant facial swelling, and complained of (C/O) pain in his right wrist and left forearm. The paramedics initiated cervical spine (C-spine) precautions, strapped him to a backboard, started oxygen (O_2) at 15 L/min via a nonrebreather mask, and started a 16-gauge IV with 0.9% normal saline (NS). His vital signs (VS) were 120/75, 125, 36, Sao_2 94%. On arrival to the local emergency department (ED) 5 minutes later his VS were 110/62, 110 regular, 28 to 32 and shallow, Sao_2 99%. An additional 16-gauge IV was inserted and the following labs were drawn: CBC, type and crossmatch (T&C), complete metabolic panel (CMP), PT/PTT INR, and alcohol (ETOH) level.

The trauma physician completed a head-to-toe assessment and found the following: Obeys commands, responds to voice but not oriented to time or place. Generalized facial edema with full-thickness 2-cm cheek laceration and bilateral mandibular depressed fractures. Blood behind left tympanic membrane (TM), edema with slight discoloration over left mastoid process. Clear drainage coming from the left nare. Mid to upper chest contusions without crepitus, breath sounds clear. Abdomen slightly firm, but not tender. Catheterized for 500 ml clear yellow urine; negative for blood, glucose, ketones. Positive deformity of right wrist and diffuse tenderness of left lower forearm.

1. On arrival, S.B. had slight discoloration over the left mastoid process, blood behind the left TM, and drainage from the nose. What is the significance of these findings?

2. S.B.'s skull x-ray study was negative for basilar skull fracture (BSF). How significant is this finding?

3. What are the typical signs and symptoms (S/S) of a BSF?

4. Identify two complications associated with BSF.

5. The term *raccoon eyes* is frequently used when describing someone who has a BSF. Explain the term *raccoon eyes*.

6. What is the most reliable diagnostic indicator for BSF?

7. How would you test S.B. for evidence of cerebrospinal fluid (CSF) leakage?

8. Identify the most serious complication of BSF.

9. What are the symptoms of a posterior fossa fracture (fracture of temporal petrous bone)?

10. S.B. is suspected of having a BSF. Why don't you want to place a nasogastric tube (NGT) in S.B.?

11. What is the treatment strategy for a BSF with a *limited* CSF leak?

chapter 7

Endocrine Disorders

Case Study 76

Scenario

You are working as an RN in a large women's clinic. Y.L., a 24-year-old Asian woman, arrives for her regularly scheduled obstetric appointment. She is in her 26th week of pregnancy and is a primigravida. After examining the patient, the nurse-midwife tells you to schedule Y.L. for a 50-g glucose challenge. You review Y.L.'s chart and note she is 5'3" and weighs 143 pounds, and her prepregnancy body mass index (BMI) is 25. Her father has type 2 diabetes mellitus (DM), and both paternal grandparents had type 2 DM. You enter the room to talk to Y.L.

1. You instruct Y.L. to drink a 50-g solution of glucose and have her blood drawn 1 hour after ingesting the solution. What is the purpose of a 50-g glucose challenge?

2. The results came back from the lab. Y.L.'s blood glucose was 151 mg/dl. What does this mean?

Based on the elevated screening test, Y.L. was scheduled for a 100-g glucose load. The lab results are as follows:

Time of Test	Patient Value	Normal Value
Fasting	101 mg/dl	<95 mg/dl
1 hour	193 mg/dl	<180 mg/dl
2 hour	132 mg/dl	<155 mg/dl
3 hour	111 mg/dl	<140 mg/dl

3. Y.L. had an elevated fasting and 1-hour test and was diagnosed with gestational diabetes mellitus (GDM). What is GDM?

4. List five risk factors for GDM. Place a star next to those risk factors that Y.L. has.

CASE STUDY PROGRESS
You schedule Y.L. with the dietitian later that same day because medical nutrition therapy (MNT) is the primary treatment for the management of GDM. She is also scheduled to meet with other members of the DM management team later in the week.

5. During the appointment with the dietitian, Y.L. gives a diet history that is high in noodles and rice with little protein. She informs the dietitian she is lactose intolerant but can have dairy products occasionally in small portions. Is it important that Y.L. take a calcium supplement along with her prenatal vitamins?

6. What is the goal of MNT?

7. Why is the MNT for a person with GDM higher in fat and protein?

8. Everyone's body metabolizes foods in different ways; however, no woman with GDM can metabolize concentrated simple sugars without a sharp rise in blood glucose. Name five examples of simple sugars.

9. Complex carbohydrates (CHO) do not cause a rapid rise in blood glucose when eaten in small amounts. Identify five foods from this group.

10. Y.L. was instructed to monitor her fasting blood glucose (FBG) first thing in the morning and 2 hours after every meal. What are the purposes of this request?

11. Y.L. was instructed to complete ketone testing using the first–voided urine in the morning. What is the rationale for this request?

Case Study **77**

Scenario

Y.L. makes an appointment to come to the clinic where you are employed. She has been complaining of (C/O) chronic fatigue, increased thirst, constant hunger, and frequent urination. She denies any pain, burning, or low-back pain on urination. She tells you she has a vaginal yeast infection that she has treated numerous times with over-the-counter (OTC) medication. She admits to starting smoking since going back to work full time as a clerk in a loan company. She also complains of having difficulty reading numbers and reports making frequent mistakes. She says, "By the time I get home, and make supper for my family, then put my child to bed, I am too tired to exercise." She reports her feet hurt; they often "burn or feel like there are pins in them." She reports that, after her delivery, she went back to her traditional eating pattern, which is high in carbohydrates (CHO).

In reviewing Y.L.'s chart, you notice she has not been seen since the delivery of her child 6 years ago. She has gained considerable weight; her current weight is 173 pounds. Today, her blood pressure (BP) is 152/97 mm Hg, and her plasma glucose is 291 mg/dl. Her primary care provider (PCP) orders the following labs: urinalysis (UA), hemoglobin A1c (Hb A_{1c}), fasting complete metabolic panel (CMP), CBC, fasting lipid profile, and glomerular filtration rate (GFR). The lab values are as follows: fasting glucose 184 mg/dl, Hb A_{1c} 10.4, UA +glucose, −ketones, cholesterol 256 mg/dl, triglycerides 346 mg/dl, LDL 155 mg/dl, HDL 32 mg/dl, ratio 8.0. A subsequent fasting glucose is also elevated, and Y.L. is diagnosed with type 2 diabetes mellitus (DM).

After meeting with Y.L. and discussing management therapies, the PCP decides to start multiple-dose injection (MDI) insulin therapy and have the patient count CHO. Y.L. is scheduled for education classes and is to work with the diabetes team to get her blood glucose under control.

1. Identify the three methods used to diagnose DM.

2. Identify three functions of insulin.

3. Insulin's main action is to lower blood glucose levels. Several hormones produced in the body inhibit the effects of insulin. Identify three.

4. Y.L. was started on lispro (Humalog) and glargine (Lantus) insulin with CHO counting. What is the most important point to make when teaching the patient about glargine?

5. Because Y.L. has been on regular insulin in the past, you want to ensure she understands the difference between regular and lispro. What is the most significant difference between these two insulins?

6. What is the peak time and duration for lispro insulin?

7. Y.L. wants to know why she can't take NPH and regular insulin. She is more familiar with them and has taken them in the past. Explain the advantages of glargine and lispro over NPH and regular insulins.

8. Y.L.'s culture prefers foods high in CHO. What is CHO counting, and why would this method work well for Y.L.?

9. Which of the symptoms that Y.L. reported today led you to believe she has some form of neuropathy?

10. What findings in Y.L.'s history place her at increased risk for the development of other forms of neuropathy?

11. What are some changes that Y.L. can make to reduce the risk or slow the progression of both macrovascular and microvascular disease?

12. Y.L. is enrolled in a smoking cessation class. Why is it so important that she stop smoking?

Case Study **78**

Name _____ **Class/Group** _____ **Date** _____
Group Members _____
INSTRUCTIONS All questions apply to this case study. Your responses should be brief and to the point. When asked to provide several answers, list them in order of priority or significance. Do not assume information that is not provided. Please print or write clearly. If your response is not legible, it will be marked as ? and you will need to rewrite it.

Scenario

You graduated 3 months ago and are working with a home care agency. Included in your caseload is J.S., a 60-year-old man suffering from chronic obstructive pulmonary disease (COPD) related to (R/T) cigarette smoking. He has been on home oxygen, 2 L oxygen by nasal cannula (O_2/NC), for several years. Approximately 10 months ago, he was started on chronic oral steroid therapy. Medications include ipratropium-albuterol (Combivent) inhaler, formoterol (Foradil) inhaler, dexamethasone (Decadron), digoxin, and furosemide (Lasix). On the way to J.S.'s home, you make a mental note to check him for signs and symptoms (S/S) of Cushing's syndrome.

1. Differentiate between Cushing's syndrome and Cushing's disease.

2. Your assessment includes the following findings. Determine whether the findings are attributable to J.S.'s COPD or possible Cushing's syndrome. Place an "L" beside the symptoms consistent with lung disease and a "C" next to those consistent with Cushing's syndrome.

____ 1. Barrel chest
____ 2. Full-looking face ("moon facies")
____ 3. Blood pressure (BP) 180/94 mm Hg
____ 4. Pursed-lip breathing, especially when patient is stressed
____ 5. Striae over trunk and thighs
____ 6. Bruising on both arms
____ 7. Acne
____ 8. Diminished breath sounds throughout lungs
____ 9. Truncal obesity with supraclavicular and posterior upper back fat and thin extremities

3. You inform the physician of the patient's S/S. The physician believes J.S. has developed Cushing's syndrome and decides to change his prescription from dexamethasone to prednisone given on alternate days. Explain the rationale for this change.

4. Identify possible consequences of suddenly stopping the dexamethasone therapy.

5. Cushing's syndrome can affect memory. Patients can easily forget what medications have been taken, especially when there are several different drugs and some are taken on alternating days. List at least three ways you can help J.S. remember to take his pills as prescribed.

6. J.S. states that his appetite has increased but he is losing weight. He reports trying to eat, but he gets short of breath (SOB) and cannot eat any more. How would you address this problem?

7. You advise J.S. to take his prednisone in the morning with food. You ask him a series of questions R/T possible gastric discomfort, vision, and joint pain. Discuss the rationale for your line of questioning.

8. Differentiate between the glucocorticoid and mineralocorticoid effects of prednisone.

9. How would your assessment change if J.S. were taking a glucocorticoid that also has significant mineralocorticoid activity?

10. Review J.S.'s list of medications. Based on what you know about the side effects of loop diuretics and steroids, discuss the potential problem of administering these in combination with digoxin.

11. Realizing that patients like J.S. are susceptible to all types of infections, you write guidelines to prevent infection. Identify four major points that these guidelines will include.

Case Study **79**

Name _____ **Class/Group** _____ **Date** _____
Group Members _____

INSTRUCTIONS All questions apply to this case study. Your responses should be brief and to the point. When asked to provide several answers, list them in order of priority or significance. Do not assume information that is not provided. Please print or write clearly. If your response is not legible, it will be marked as ? and you will need to rewrite it.

Scenario

You are working in a community outpatient clinic where you perform the intake assessment on R.M., a 38-year-old woman who is attending graduate school and is very sedentary. Her chief complaint (C/C) is overwhelming fatigue that is not relieved by rest. She is so exhausted that she has difficulty walking to classes and trouble concentrating when studying. Her face looks puffy, and her skin is dry and pale. She complains of (C/O) generalized body aches and pains with frequent muscle cramps and constipation. You notice she is dressed inappropriately warm for the weather. Initial vital signs (VS) were 142/84, 52, 12, 96.8°F.

1. Compare her VS with those of a healthy person her same age.

2. List eight general questions you might ask R.M. to get a "ball park" idea of what is going on with her.

3. You know that potential causes for some of R.M.'s symptoms include depression, hypothyroidism, anemia, cardiac disease, fluid and electrolyte imbalance, and allergies. As part of your screening procedures, describe how you would begin to investigate which of these conditions probably do *not* account for R.M.'s symptoms.

CASE STUDY PROGRESS
R.M. is slightly bradycardic but you find no obvious irregularities in her cardiopulmonary assessment.

4. Unnecessary diagnostic tests are expensive. What tests do you think would be the most important for R.M., and why?

CASE STUDY PROGRESS
R.M.'s thyroid-stimulating hormone (TSH) comes back 20.9 IU/L; the family nurse practitioner diagnoses R.M. with hypothyroidism and places her on thyroid replacement therapy.

5. The practitioner prescribes levothyroxine (Synthroid) 1.7 mcg/kg body weight/day. At this time, R.M. weighs 130 pounds. What should be her daily dose of levothyroxine in milligrams? How would her prescription read?

✳**Note:** *Until recently, micrograms were alternately written as µg or mcg on prescriptions. These are still acceptable for calculations. However, Joint Commission standards have changed, and these units of measure are no longer acceptable on prescriptions.*

6. R.M.'s TSH level is increased. Explain the relationship between these laboratory results and hypothyroidism.

7. What patient teaching needs will you review with R.M. before she leaves? Remember medication issues.

8. Why would you want to obtain a complete drug history on R.M.?

9. What general teaching issues would you address with R.M.?

10. R.M. wonders whether she should take iodine supplements if she decreases her salt intake. She recognizes that salt is a significant source of iodine in her part of the country. What would you explain to her?

11. What should you teach R.M. regarding prevention of myxedema coma?

✳ **Note:** *TSH should be checked annually once R.M. is stable on medication.*

12. Before R.M. leaves the clinic, she asks how she will know whether the medication is "doing its job." Outline simple expected outcomes for R.M.

13. Several weeks later, R.M. calls the clinic stating she can't remember whether she took her thyroid medication. What additional data should you obtain, and how would you advise her?

14. Under what circumstances should R.M. hold the drug or call the clinic?

CASE STUDY PROGRESS

R.M. comes in 2 months later for a follow-up (F/U) visit. You can't believe she is the same person. She looks and walks as if she were 10 years younger. Her skin appears more radiant, and her hair looks much healthier. "You can't believe how different I'm feeling," she says. "I didn't know how bad off I was; I'm starting to live again."

For more information, contact:

American Thyroid Association: *http://www.thyroid.org*

National Library of Medicine: *http://www.nlm.nih.gov*

Thyroid Foundation of America: *http:/www.allthyroid.org*

Case Study **80**

Scenario

K.B. is an 80-year-old man admitted to the hospital following a 5-day episode of the "flu" with complaints of (C/O) dyspnea on exertion (DOE), palpitations, chest pain, insomnia, and fatigue. His past medical history (PMH) includes heart failure (HF) and hypertension (HTN) requiring antihypertensive medications (he states that he has not been taking these medications on a regular basis). K.B. was diagnosed with Graves' disease 6 months ago and was placed on methimazole (Tapazole) 15 mg/day PO. Assessment findings are as follows: height 5'8", weight 130 pounds; appears anxious and restless; loud heart sounds; vital signs (VS): 150/90, 104 irregular, 20, 100.2°F; 1+ pitting edema noted in bilateral lower extremities; diminished breath sounds with fine crackles in the posterior bases. K.B. begins to cry when he tells you he recently lost his wife; you notice someone has punched several more holes in his belt so he could tighten it. Laboratory findings are Hgb 11.8 g/dl, Hct 36%, erythrocyte sedimentation rate (ESR) 48 mm/hr, Na 141 mmol/L, K 4.7 mmol/L, Cl 101 mmol/L, BUN 33 mg/dl, creatinine 1.9 mg/dl, T_4 14.0 mcg/dl, T_3 230 ng/dl.

1. Of the physical assessment and laboratory findings, which represent manifestations of hypermetabolism?

2. What additional subjective and objective data would you gather from someone with Graves' disease?

3. After morning rounds, the physician leaves the following orders: propranolol (Inderal) 20 mg PO q6h, dexamethasone (Decadron) 10 mg IV q6h, verapamil (Calan SR) 120 mg/day PO, diet as tolerated, STAT ECG, up ad lib. Which of the orders would you question and why?

4. Develop four priority problems related to K.B.'s care.

5. Later on your shift, you note that K.B. is extremely restless and is disoriented to person, place, and time. VS are 104/62, 180 and irregular, 32 and labored, 104° F. His ECG shows atrial fibrillation (A-fib). What do these findings indicate?

6. What would you do first?

CASE STUDY PROGRESS

K.B. is in thyroid crisis. The physician orders the following labs STAT: arterial blood gases (ABGs). He also orders digoxin (Lanoxin) 0.5 mg IV push (IVP) now and 0.250 mg IVP q8h × 2 doses; IV of D₅W at 100 ml/hr; increase methimazole to 15 mg PO q6h; Lugol's solution (strong iodine) 10 drops PO tid mixed in water or juice to start 1 hour after the first methimazole dose; hydrocortisone (HydroCort) 50 mg IVP q6h; cardiac monitor; absolute bed rest; acetaminophen (Tylenol) 650 mg PO q6h prn for temperature over 100° F.

�֍ **7.** Identify four measures that would be essential in caring for K.B.

8. Identify two possible factors that may have either precipitated or contributed to K.B.'s thyroid storm.

9. Before discharge, the physician discusses two treatment options with K.B. and his family: radioactive iodine (RAI) therapy using ^{131}I, and subtotal thyroidectomy. K.B. is fearful of radiation treatment and asks you for your opinion. How would you respond?

10. K.B. decides to receive ^{131}I. During pretreatment instructions, the family asks if he will be radioactive and what precautions they should take. Outline important guidelines for instructing K.B. and his family on home precautions.

11. Discuss how your discharge teaching instructions will differ from those you would give to someone following a subtotal thyroidectomy.

Case Study **81**

Name _____ Class/Group _____ Date _____
Group Members _____
INSTRUCTIONS All questions apply to this case study. Your responses should be brief and to the point. When asked to provide several answers, list them in order of priority or significance. Do not assume information that is not provided. Please print or write clearly. If your response is not legible, it will be marked as ? and you will need to rewrite it.

Scenario

You are working on an oncology unit and will be receiving a patient from the recovery room. The postanesthesia care unit (PACU) nurse calls and gives the following report: C.P. is a 50-year-old woman with a subtotal thyroidectomy for multinodular goiter and left superior and right inferior parathyroidectomy because of adenoma. The estimated blood loss (EBL) was 25 ml. Vital signs (VS) are 130/82, 80 to 90, 20, Sao_2 94% on room air. She has a peripheral IV of D_5.45NS with 20 mEq KCl and 10 mEq calcium gluconate infusing at 100 ml/hr. She has received a total of 50 mg meperidine IV push (IVP), and she remains awake, alert, and oriented (AAO). C.P.'s past medical history (PMH) includes total abdominal hysterectomy (TAH) for fibroids and low-level radiation treatments to the neck 38 years ago for eczema. Her medications include estradiol, lovastatin, and levothyroxine. Both parents are living; her father had a myocardial infarction (MI) at 70 years of age; her mother has hypothyroidism but never had thyroid tumors. Preoperative laboratory findings are Ca 11.2 mg/dl, phosphorus 2.4 mg/dl, Cl 106 mmol/L, alkaline phosphatase 112 units/L, elevated PTH and thyroid-stimulating hormone (TSH) levels, creatinine 1.4 mg/dl.

1. What additional data should you obtain from the recovery room nurse?

2. What preparations will you make before C.P. arrives?

3. You receive C.P. from the recovery room. How will you focus your initial assessment, and why?

4. During your initial assessment, you document negative Chvostek's and Trousseau's signs. Describe data that would support this conclusion.

5. Identify the major risk factor that may have contributed to the development of parathyroid adenoma in C.P.

�֍ 6. Identify four actions you should include in the postoperative care of C.P. Anticipate and monitor for signs of:

7. Identify measures that reduce the risk for postoperative swelling.

8. After surgery, C.P.'s thyroid hormone levels were elevated and the physician ordered propranolol 80 mg ER (extended-release) tabs for "surgically induced thyrotoxicosis." Is this reaction expected following parathyroid surgery or did something go wrong during surgery? Explain.

9. Eighteen hours after surgery, C.P. calls you into her room complaining of (C/O) numbness around her mouth and tingling at the tips of her fingers. She appears restless but is AAO. Realizing that C.P. may be experiencing hypocalcemia, you notify the physician. What should you do in the interim before the physician returns your call?

CASE STUDY PROGRESS

C.P. is given supplemental calcium gluconate and recovers without further complications. C.P. is started on calcium carbonate bid, is given a F/U (follow-up) appointment in 3 weeks, and is discharged 24 hours postoperatively.

Case Study **82**

Scenario

You work in a diabetes mellitus (DM) treatment center located in a large teaching hospital. The first patient you meet is K.W., a 40-year-old Hispanic female, who was seen 2 years ago with symptoms of severe fatigue and blurred vision. She thought this was due to working long hours at a computer. The physician who examined her told her she had "borderline diabetes," gave her a 1200-calorie diet, and told her to lose weight. Her records from that visit indicate the following: weight 205 pounds, height 5'4", blood pressure (BP) 140/90 mm Hg, urine normal, and fasting glucose 118 mg/dl.

1. The correct term for "borderline diabetes" is either *impaired fasting glucose* (IFG) or *impaired glucose tolerance* (IGT); another term commonly used now is *prediabetes*. How would you explain the term *borderline diabetes* to K.W.?

2. What are the criteria for the diagnosis of IFG or IGT?

3. What laboratory value indicated that K.W. had IFG or prediabetes?

4. What recommendations would you have made to K.W. to minimize her risk of developing DM in the future?

CASE STUDY PROGRESS

K.W. did not think she had a problem and ignored the physician's advice. Three days ago K.W. went to see the physician after a 1-month history of frequent urination, thirst, fatigue, and some burning and tingling in her feet. She smokes and does not exercise. Her diet is mostly fast foods, and the foods cooked at home are high in starch and fat. Because of her work schedule, her mealtimes vary from day to day. Her family history includes her father dying of myocardial infarction (MI) in his 40s and her mother suffering from DM and HTN.

The labs from her physician's visit are as follows: weight 215 pounds, random glucose 210 mg/dl, next day fasting glucose 135 mg/dl, Hb A$_{1c}$ 9.5%, cholesterol 310 mg/dl, triglycerides 300 mg/dl, HDL 25 mg/dl, LDL 160 mg/dl, ratio 12.4, creatinine 0.9 mg/dl, body mass index (BMI) 37.6, BP 160/96 mm Hg. She is diagnosed with type 2 DM and is started on metformin for her diabetes, lisinopril for her HTN, and simvastatin for her hyperlipidemia. She is referred to the diabetes treatment center for comprehensive education.

5. What laboratory values are now diagnostic for type 2 DM?

CASE STUDY PROGRESS

Your educational materials cover 4 basic areas: medical nutrition therapy (MNT), exercise, glucose monitoring, and pharmacotherapy.

6. Identify important points to be covered under MNT.

7. Identify important content to be included under exercise. Address potential benefits, precautions, and recommendations.

8. Identify important content to be included under glucose monitoring.

9. Identify important content to be included under pharmacologic therapy.

CASE STUDY PROGRESS

K.W. expresses concern over the burning and tingling in her feet. She comments, "I've heard many people with diabetes can lose their toes or even their feet." You take this opportunity to teach K.W. about neuropathy and foot care.

10. How would you educate K.W. about neuropathy?

11. No diabetic education program would be complete without addressing good foot care. Identify seven points you would include when teaching K.W. about proper diabetic foot care.

12. Given all the information in the foregoing scenario, what DM–related complication do you believe K.W. is most at risk for and why?

13. List at least three interventions for reducing K.W.'s risk for macrovascular disease.

14. K.W. states she and her husband were planning on having another child in a year to two. She wants to know how her having DM will affect this. Pregnancy in persons with DM is a complex issue. What basic information can you share with K.W. today without overwhelming her?

✳ **Note:** *The American Association of Clinical Endocrinologists (AACE) recommends an Hb A$_{1c}$ level of 6.5% or less. The ADA still recommends 7.0% or less.*

chapter 8

Immunologic Disorders

Case Study 83

Scenario

You are a nurse at a student health clinic. T.Q. comes in to your clinic and informs you of his immunodeficiency problem. He has just moved here to go to school. He gives you a letter from his attending physician, hands you a vial of gamma globulin, and asks you to give him his "shot." The letter from T.Q.'s physician states that he was diagnosed with primary immunodeficiency disease 18 years ago. He has an adequate number of B cells, but they fail to mature properly and become plasma cells or immunoglobulin. T.Q. states he has a history of chronic respiratory and gastrointestinal (GI) infections. He is maintained on 0.66 ml/kg gamma globulin IM every 3 weeks and has tolerated this well. He has no known drug allergies (NKDA). His vital signs (VS) are stable.

1. Can you honor this patient's prescription? Why or why not? How could you provide him with his injection?

2. What should you do while the physician is verifying information?

3. Once the clinic physician receives confirmation from T.Q.'s physician, he will order the gamma globulin. What questions would you ask T.Q. that would reassure you that the medication he brought was safe to administer?

4. Briefly describe the maturation cycle of the B cell.

5. What immunoglobulin deficiency does T.Q. have?

6. Before T.Q. leaves, you should assess his knowledge and give specific precautions. What should you assess, and what precautions should you give?

7. You note on T.Q.'s health record that he has not received his polio, measles, mumps, or rubella vaccines. What explanation can be given for the lack of these vaccinations?

8. T.Q. returns in 3 weeks with complaints of (C/O) a stuffy nose. What will you assess to further evaluate his stuffy nose?

9. If T.Q. is developing a sinus infection, what signs are you likely to encounter on examining him?

CASE STUDY PROGRESS

T.Q.'s nares do not appear swollen or red, although he does have some clear mucus drainage. His temperature is normal at 98.4°F. T.Q. is due for his next injection of gamma globulin.

10. Should you give the medication or ask him to return when he is no longer having nasal stuffiness? Why or why not?

11. How do primary immunodeficiencies differ from secondary immunodeficiencies?

12. What is the most common primary immunodeficiency?

13. Explain why T.Q. is at greater risk for developing infections than his classmates.

Case Study **84**

Scenario

You are working at a physician's office, and you have just taken C.Q., a 38-year-old woman, into the consultation room. C.Q. has been divorced for 5 years, has 2 daughters (ages 14 and 16), and works full time as a legal secretary. Two weeks ago she visited her physician for a routine physical examination and requested that a human immunodeficiency virus (HIV) test be performed. C.Q. stated that she was in a serious relationship, is contemplating marriage, and just wanted to make certain she was OK. No abnormalities were noted during C.Q.'s physical examination, and blood was drawn for routine blood chemistries, hematology studies, and an enzyme-linked immunosorbent assay (ELISA) test (also known as the enzyme immunoassay [EIA] test). C.Q. is at the office to receive her lab results. The physician informs you that C.Q.'s EIA was positive.

1. What is an EIA test? Does a positive EIA mean that C.Q. definitely has HIV?

2. You explain to C.Q. that one of her tests needs to be repeated and you need to draw another blood sample. Why wouldn't you tell C.Q. that her first test result was positive and that another test is needed before the diagnosis can be confirmed?

CASE STUDY PROGRESS

The physician informs you that C.Q.'s Western blot test results confirm that she is HIV positive; he requests that you be present when he talks to her. Before leaving C.Q.'s room, the physician requests that you obtain another blood sample for further testing, give C.Q. verbal and written information about local acquired immunodeficiency syndrome (AIDS) support groups, and help C.Q. call a friend to accompany her home this evening. She looks at you through her tears and states, "I can't believe it. J. is the only man I've had sex with since my divorce. He told me I had nothing to worry about. I can't believe he would do this to me."

3. C.Q.'s statement is based on 3 assumptions: (1) J. is HIV positive, (2) he intentionally withheld the information from her, and (3) he intentionally transmitted the HIV to her through unprotected sex. Based on your knowledge of HIV infection, how would you counsel C.Q.?

4. In addition to offering alternative explanations and exploring options, what is your most important role at this time?

5. Identify at least three issues related to (R/T) C.Q.'s care.

6. C.Q. has had a positive EIA test and is seropositive for HIV. Why doesn't she have signs and symptoms (S/S) of AIDS?

7. What are some of the acute signs and symptoms of an HIV infection?

8. Why is it a good idea for C.Q. to have someone she trusts transport her home this evening?

CASE STUDY PROGRESS

C.Q. gives you the name and phone number of a relative she wants you to call. You remain with her until she leaves with her relative.

9. Has C.Q.'s right to privacy been violated? Explain why or why not.

10. C.Q. returns to the office 4 days later to discuss her diagnosis. What issues will you discuss with her at this time?

11. Does C.Q. have a legal responsibility to inform J. of her HIV status?

CASE STUDY PROGRESS

Two weeks later C.Q. visits the office and asks to speak to you in private. She thanks you for talking to her the day she received the news of her diagnosis. She pulls a gun from her purse and states, "I was going to go out into the waiting room and blow J. away, because I thought he was cheating on me." She tells you that J. confessed to her he was afraid to tell her about his hemophilia because she might leave him. J. was tested for HIV at regular intervals and his last HIV test, 6 months ago, had been negative. J. was retested, and this test was positive for HIV. J.'s doctor discussed the possibility of transmission through recombinant factor VIII products. C.Q. tells you that they are going to get married and invites you to the wedding. She stops at the door and says, "At least we won't have to worry about safe sex with each other!"

Case Study **85**

Scenario

J.P., a 56-year-old man, developed a severe viral infection and suffered fatigue, fever, and myalgia. Although he recovered from the acute episode, J.P. never quite regained his normal activity level. Six months later, J.P. continues to find it difficult to work a 10-hour day as a brick mason, so he returns to his physician. Diagnostic studies reveal heart failure (HF) related to (R/T) postviral cardiomyopathy.

Following medical management with metoprolol (Toprol XL) and furosemide (Lasix), his condition stabilizes and he returns to work, but his attendance is erratic. J.P.'s condition gradually deteriorates. Sixteen months later he is readmitted to the hospital complaining of (C/O) dyspnea with minimal exertion, fatigue, orthopnea, chest pain, anorexia, and feelings of abdominal fullness. He has 1+ peripheral edema and is diaphoretic. Further studies reveal that J.P. has cardiac dilation, moderate to gross ventricular hypertrophy, and poor systolic ejection fraction (EF 17%), consistent with severe congestive cardiomyopathy. Because J.P.'s only other health problem is mild hypertension (HTN), heart transplant evaluation is recommended. J.P. and his wife discuss his prognosis, and he agrees to an evaluation for possible heart transplantation.

1. If J.P. is accepted for cardiac transplantation, what data will be collected in addition to his past medical history (PMH), current diagnostic findings, and cardiac evaluation?

2. What criteria does J.P. meet that will make him eligible for cardiac transplantation?

3. Identify five contraindications for cardiac transplant.

4. J.P. is accepted for cardiac transplant and placed on the waiting list. What fears or concerns may J.P. experience during this waiting period?

CASE STUDY PROGRESS

J.P. receives a phone call to report to the hospital immediately because a donor heart has become available.

5. What compatibility tests are performed to determine eligibility for transplantation and to ensure as close a match as possible?

6. As the nurse on the transplant unit, how can you best help J.P. prepare for his heart transplant?

CASE STUDY PROGRESS

J.P.'s surgery and recovery are uncomplicated, and he is sent home and referred to cardiac rehabilitation after adjustment of his immunosuppression therapy and appropriate teaching. J.P. is readmitted for low-grade fever and dyspnea 6 weeks after surgery. Cardiac biopsies demonstrate moderate acute rejection.

7. What is the etiology of acute rejection, and how does it differ from chronic rejection?

8. The nurse can anticipate that prompt immunosuppressive therapy will be instituted using what drugs? How do these alter the rejection process?

✳ **9.** What is the most important intervention for J.P. at this time, and why?

CASE STUDY PROGRESS

J.P. responds positively to steroid therapy and is released to home after 5 days. J.P. is again admitted to the hospital with renewed C/O of dyspnea, low-grade fever, and ankle swelling 7 months later. Both J.P. and his wife are anxious and fearful.

10. Explain what may be happening to J.P. physiologically.

11. How will treatment for this episode of graft rejection differ from treatment for his earlier episode of rejection?

12. J.P.'s prognosis for the future will depend on what factors?

Case Study **86**

Name _____ **Class/Group** _____ **Date** _____
Group Members _____
INSTRUCTIONS All questions apply to this case study. Your responses should be brief and to the point. When asked
to provide several answers, list them in order of priority or significance. Do not assume information that is not provided.
Please print or write clearly. If your response is not legible, it will be marked as ? and you will need to rewrite it.

Scenario

W.V. is a 57-year-old man who lives with his wife and 2 teenage sons. W.V. developed chronic kidney
disease 20 years ago after acute kidney disease related to (R/T) phenacetin use. (W.V. took phenacetin
since his early 20s for migraine headaches. Large doses of phenacetin over the years can cause
analgesic-induced nephropathy. This drug has subsequently been removed from the market.) W.V. was
initially placed on hemodialysis for 5 years before receiving a cadaveric transplant, or cadaver kidney.
He recovered without complications, and his serum laboratory values returned to normal. He was
placed on triple immunosuppression therapy, including prednisone, cyclosporin, and mycophenolate
(CellCept) and was discharged to home. W.V. returned to work 3 weeks later.

Today W.V. reports to his physician for routine follow-up (F/U). His vital signs (VS) are 148/92, 88,
24, 99.2° F. His lab data reveal the following: serum creatinine 1.2 mg/dl, BUN 22 mg/dl, normal serum
electrolytes. W.V. has gained 5 pounds since discharge from the hospital.

1. What histocompatibility studies are generally performed before renal transplant, and why
are they important?

2. By what criteria is W.V. considered a good candidate for renal transplantation?

3. If W.V.'s kidney is producing sufficient urine and he is feeling well, why is it necessary to
monitor his laboratory data?

4. What is the possible significance of W.V.'s current blood pressure (BP)?

5. How does the drug mycophenolate protect W.V.'s kidney from rejection, and what are the most important side effects of this drug that W.V. must be taught to monitor?

6. How will W.V. know whether he is experiencing organ rejection?

7. If W.V. begins to reject his kidney, how would the rejection be classified, and what signs and symptoms (S/S) would most likely be present?

8. Identify at least four ways that W.V. might experience difficulty adjusting to his organ transplant.

9. How can you best support W.V. and his family?

10. Why is it necessary for W.V. to be concerned about infection?

Case Study **87**

Scenario

K.D. is a 36-year-old gay professional man who has been human immunodeficiency virus (HIV) positive
for 6 years. Until recently, he demonstrated no signs and symptoms (S/S) of acquired immunodeficiency
syndrome (AIDS). The appearance of purplish spots on his neck and arms persuaded him to make an
appointment with his physician. When he arrives at the physician's office, the nurse performs a brief
assessment. His vital signs (VS) are 138/86, 100, 30, 100.8°F. K.D. states that he has been feeling
fatigued for several months and is experiencing occasional night sweats, but he also has been working
long hours, has skipped meals, and has been particularly stressed over a project at work. K.D.'s physical examination is within normal limits (WNL) except for his rapid heart rate and respirations, low-grade
fever, and skin lesions. The doctor orders a chest x-ray (CXR), CBC, lymphocyte studies, ultra viral load,
Cytomegalovirus (CMV) assay, and a PPD (purified protein derivative) test. K.D. made an appointment
to return in 5 days to discuss the results of his tests.

Over the next 2 weeks, K.D. develops a fever of 101°F, nonproductive cough, and increasing shortness of breath (SOB). Late one night he becomes acutely SOB, so his roommate, J.F., takes him to the
emergency department (ED) where he is subsequently admitted to the hospital with probable *Pneu-
mocystis carinii* pneumonia (PCP). Bronchoalveolar lavage examined under light microscopy confirms
the diagnosis. K.D.'s admission WBC and lymphocyte studies demonstrate an increased pattern of
immunodeficiency compared with earlier studies. K.D. is placed on nasal oxygen, IV fluids, and IV
trimethoprim-sulfamethoxazole (Septra, Bactrim).

1. What is PCP?

2. What is the significance of the purplish spots over K.D.'s neck and arms?

3. Identify four problems for K.D.

4. What precautions will you need to use when caring for K.D.?

❇ 5. What will be the focus of your ongoing assessment? (List three.)

6. What major side effects of his antibiotic should you monitor K.D. for?

7. Differentiate between HIV–positive status and AIDS.

8. Why is K.D.'s development of PCP of particular importance in light of his HIV status?

9. K.D. has been seropositive for several years, yet he has been asymptomatic for AIDS. What factors may have influenced K.D.'s development of PCP?

CASE STUDY PROGRESS
K.D. is responding well to treatment, and plans are being made for discharge. He will be started on standard therapy, with follow-up (F/U) on an outpatient basis. Because "standard therapy" changes in response to developments in clinical research, you will have to look up the most recent recommended treatment.

10. K.D. was taught about disease transmission and safer sex and encouraged to maintain moderate exercise, rest, and dietary habits when he was first diagnosed as HIV positive. Give at least four additional topics that should be discussed with K.D. before he goes home.

11. What laboratory data will most likely be monitored on K.D. in the future?

12. List at least five other opportunistic infections that K.D. is at risk for developing.

For additional information, check the following resources:
The Body: The Complete HIV/AIDS Resource: *http://www.thebody.com*
National Institute of Allergy and Infectious Diseases: *http://www.niaid.nih.gov*

Case Study **88**

Name _____ Class/Group_____ Date _____
Group Members _____

INSTRUCTIONS All questions apply to this case study. Your responses should be brief and to the point. When asked to provide several answers, list them in order of priority or significance. Do not assume information that is not provided. Please print or write clearly. If your response is not legible, it will be marked as ? and you will need to rewrite it.

Scenario

D.W. is a 23-year-old married woman with 3 children under 5 years old. She came to her physician 2 years ago with vague complaints of (C/O) intermittent fatigue, joint pain, low-grade fever, and unintentional weight loss.

Her physician noted small patchy areas of vitiligo and a scaly rash across her nose, cheeks, back, and chest at that time. Laboratory studies revealed that D.W. had a positive antinuclear antibody (ANA) titer, positive dsDNA (positive lupus erythematosus), positive anti-Sm (antismooth muscle antibody), elevated C-reactive protein (CRP) and erythrocyte sedimentation rate (ESR), and decreased C3 and C4 serum complement. Joint x-ray films demonstrated joint swelling without joint erosion. D.W. was subsequently diagnosed with systemic lupus erythematosus (SLE). She was initially treated with sulindac 200 mg PO bid, prednisone 20 mg/day PO, bed rest, and ice packs. She was counseled regarding her condition and advised to balance rest and activity, eat a well-balanced diet, use strategies to reduce stress, and avoid direct sunlight. D.W. responded well to treatment, the steroid was tapered and discontinued, and she was told she could report for follow-up (F/U) every 6 months unless her symptoms became acute. D.W. resumed her job in environmental services at a large geriatric facility.

1. What is the significance of each of D.W.'s laboratory findings?

2. Given that most tests are nonspecific, how is SLE diagnosed?

3. What priority problems need to be addressed with D.W.?

CASE STUDY PROGRESS

Eighteen months after diagnosis, D.W. seeks out her physician because of puffy hands and feet and increased fatigue. D.W. reports that she has been working longer hours because of the absence of 2 of her fellow workers. Her chem 8 reveals that her BUN and creatinine are slightly elevated, and her urinalysis (UA) shows 2+ protein and 1+ RBCs.

4. Of what significance are these findings, and what is the relationship of such findings to D.W.'s diagnosis of SLE?

5. How will D.W.'s treatment and care plan likely change?

CASE STUDY PROGRESS

D.W. is seen in the immunology clinic twice monthly during the next 3 months. Although her condition does not worsen, her BUN and creatinine remain elevated. While at work one afternoon, D.W. begins to feel dizzy and develops a severe headache. She reports to her supervisor, who has her lie down. When D.W. starts to become disoriented, her supervisor calls 911, and D.W. is taken to the hospital. D.W. is admitted for probable lupus cerebritis related to (R/T) acute exacerbation of her disease.

6. What preventive measures should be instituted to protect D.W. at this time?

7. What additional problems indicative of central nervous system (CNS) involvement R/T SLE should D.W. be assessed for?

CASE STUDY PROGRESS

The physician ordered methylprednisolone and plasmapheresis.

8. What major complications associated with immunosuppression therapy will D.W. have to be monitored for?

9. What does plasmapheresis do, and why might it reduce the signs and symptoms (S/S) associated with SLE?

10. What data would support the assumption that D.W.'s condition is stabilizing?

11. Identify at least five topics that D.W. must be taught before she is discharged that may help her lead as normal a life as possible.

12. You note that D.W.'s husband is visiting her this afternoon. You enter the room to ask whether they have any questions. D.W.'s husband states, "I have tried to tell her that she cannot go back to work. Sure, we need the money, but the kids and I need her more. I'm afraid that this lupus has weakened her whole body and it will kill her if she goes back to work. Is that right?" How should you respond to his concerns?

Additional information on SLE can be found through the following resources:

Lupus Foundation of America, Inc.: *http://www.lupus.org*

MedlinePlus: *http://www.nlm.nih.gov/medlineplus/lupus.html*

National Institute of Arthritis and Musculoskeletal and Skin Diseases: *http://www.niams.nih.gov*

Bonus Project

Locate and print a patient education handout on SLE in both English and Spanish. Attach it to this assignment.

Oncologic and Hematologic Disorders

Case Study 89

Name _____ Class/Group _____ Date _____
Group Members _____
INSTRUCTIONS All questions apply to this case study. Your responses should be brief and to the point. When asked
to provide several answers, list them in order of priority or significance. Do not assume information that is not provided.
Please print or write clearly. If your response is not legible, it will be marked as ? and you will need to rewrite it.

Scenario

You are a home health nurse who has been seeing P.C., who was diagnosed with lung cancer approximately 1 year ago. Her provider recently informed her that her cancer is no longer treatable; the focus of her treatment will change from curative measures to symptom relief. She is confused and somewhat angry with her provider. She vaguely remembers the term *palliative treatment* when discussing her situation with her provider but doesn't know what it means.

1. How would you describe palliative treatment?

CASE STUDY PROGRESS

P.C. confides that she always felt that she might not survive her illness, but has never formally written down her wishes concerning what types of treatment she would or would not want. You advise her to complete an advance directive and/or living will or to complete a medical durable power of attorney and/or a surrogate decision maker form. In current practice, it is very likely that a part of the home health intake process will be completion of a Physicians Order on Life Sustaining Treatments (POLST) Paradigm form.

2.   What is the purpose of these documents?

3.   What health care decisions are considered in these documents?

4.   How are advance directives and living wills formalized?

5.   P.C. states she is confused and has mixed feelings about her health care wishes right now. She asks, "If I fill out this form, can I change my mind down the road?" How should you answer this question?

6. You inform P.C. that you will help with symptomatic control of her illness. What areas will you focus on, and what question would you ask P.C.?

7. As P.C. becomes more frail and incoherent, what treatment will be given?

Case Study **90**

Name _____ Class/Group _____ Date _____
Group Members _____

INSTRUCTIONS All questions apply to this case study. Your responses should be brief and to the point. When asked to provide several answers, list them in order of priority or significance. Do not assume information that is not provided. Please print or write clearly. If your response is not legible, it will be marked as ? and you will need to rewrite it.

Scenario

G.C. is a 78-year-old widow who relies on her late husband's Social Security income for all her expenses. Over the past few years, G.C. has eaten less and less meat because of her financial situation and the trouble of preparing a meal "just for me." She also has medicines to buy for the treatment of hypertension (HTN) and arthritis. Over the past 2 to 3 months, she has felt increasingly tired, despite sleeping well at night. When she goes to the senior clinic, the nurse practitioner orders blood work. The lab results are as follows: WBC 7.6 thou/cmm, Hct 27.3%, Hgb 8.3 mg/dl, platelets 151 thou/cmm. RBC indices are mean corpuscular volume (MCV) 65 cmm, mean corpuscular hemoglobin (MCH) 31.6 pg, MCH concentration (MCHC) 35.1%, red cell distribution width (RDW) 15.6%. Other results were iron (Fe) 30 mcg/dl, total iron-binding capacity (TIBC) 422 mcg/dl, ferritin 8 mg/dl, vitamin B_{12} 414 pg/ml, folate 188 ng/ml. Chem 14 is within normal limits (WNL). Stool guaiac test is negative.

1. Which lab values are normal, and which are abnormal?

2. Explain the significance of the abnormal results.

3. What type of anemia does G.C. have?

4. What are some causative factors for the type of anemia G.C. has?

5. Which individuals are at risk?

6. Describe some of the other signs and symptoms (S/S) of this type of anemia.

7. Discuss some of the treatment options for her disease.

8. Discuss some ideas that may help her with her meal planning.

Case Study **91**

Scenario

You are a nurse working in the local emergency department (ED) when J.B., a well-known 62-year-old
homeless alcoholic, comes in. He has a long history of tobacco use, poor diet, and no dental care.
Over the past several months he has experienced increasing shortness of breath (SOB), hoarseness,
and odynophagia. On examination he is found to have 2 left-sided cervical nodes, which are firm and
fixed. A piriform sinus mass is found on bronchoscopy. Biopsy confirms squamous cell carcinoma. The
large mass extends to and is fixed to the left true vocal cord. Chest x-ray (CXR) is normal with the
exception of changes related to chronic tobacco use. Past medical history (PMH) includes reactive
airway disease and hypertension (HTN). J.B. is scheduled for a direct laryngoscopy, total laryngectomy
with left radical neck dissection, and placement of a permanent tracheostomy.

1. Identify risk factors for head and neck cancer present in this case.

2. Name the warning signals listed on the American Cancer Society's list of warning signs of
cancer. Which of these did J.B. have? Please see the website listed at the end of this case
study for more information.

CASE STUDY PROGRESS
J.B. is initially seen with odynophagia, hoarseness, thickening in cervical nodes.

3. Describe the surgical intervention J.B. will undergo.

4. J.B. has several important postoperative needs. Identify two serious complications for which he is most at risk.

5. What type of follow-up (F/U) therapy is J.B. likely to undergo after his initial wound heals?

6. Postoperatively, J.B. requires placement of a percutaneous endoscopic gastrostomy (PEG) feeding tube because he is unable to maintain adequate nutritional intake. Discuss one problem related to each of the following: nutrition, airway maintenance, and communication.

7. J.B. has several factors that make discharge planning especially problematic. Describe three specific discharge problems, and list possible solutions.

For more information on updates for early detection of specific cancers, visit *http://www.cancer. org/docroot/PED/content/PED_2_3X_ACS_Cancer_Detection_Guidelines_36.asp?sitearea=PED.*

Case Study **92**

Scenario

R.T. is a 64-year-old man who comes to his primary care provider's (PCP's) office for a yearly examination. He initially reports having no new health problems; however, on further questioning, he admits to having developed some fatigue, abdominal bloating, and intermittent constipation. His nurse practitioner completes the examination, which includes a normal rectal exam with a stool positive for guaiac. Diagnostic studies include a CBC with differential, chem 14, and carcinoembryonic antigen (CEA). R.T. has not had a recent colonoscopy and is referred to a gastroenterologist for this procedure. A 5-cm mass found in the sigmoid colon confirms a diagnosis of adenocarcinoma of the colon. A referral is made for surgery. The pathology report describes the tumor as a Dukes' stage B, which means that the cancer has extended into the mucous layer of the colon. A metastatic work-up is negative.

1. What is a risk factor?

2. Identify six risk factors for colon cancer.

3. Discuss the American Cancer Society's recommended screening procedures related to colon cancer.

✳ **Note:** *These recommendations are based on asymptomatic individuals and may be changed based on results of screening exams.*

4. According to the American Cancer Society, what warning signs did R.T. have?

5. Discuss common early versus late signs and symptoms (S/S) found in individuals with colorectal cancer.

6. What is a CEA? How does it relate to the diagnosis of colon cancer?

7. After bowel prep, R.T. is admitted to the hospital for an exploratory laparotomy, small bowel resection, and sigmoid colectomy. List at least five major potential complications for R.T.

8. After surgery, R.T. is admitted to the surgical intensive care unit (SICU) with a large abdominal dressing. The nurse rolls R.T. side to side to remove the soiled surgical linen, and the dressing becomes saturated with a large amount of serosanguineous drainage. Would the drainage be expected after abdominal surgery? Explain.

9. Four weeks after surgery, R.T. is scheduled to begin chemotherapy. List three chemotherapy drugs used to treat adenocarcinoma of the colon.

10. Discuss some of the toxicities and side effects of these drugs.

11. Given the side effect profiles of the drugs used to treat colon cancer, develop a teaching plan for R.T.

Case Study **93**

Name _____ Class/Group_____Date _____
Group Members _____
INSTRUCTIONS All questions apply to this case study. Your responses should be brief and to the point. When asked
to provide several answers, list them in order of priority or significance. Do not assume information that is not provided.
Please print or write clearly. If your response is not legible, it will be marked as ? and you will need to rewrite it.

Scenario

M.D. is a 50-year-old woman who was notified of an abnormal screening mammogram. Diagnosis of infiltrating ductal carcinoma was made following a stereotactic needle biopsy of a 1.5 × 1.5 cm lobu-lated mass at the 3:00 position in her left breast. M.D. had a modified radical mastectomy with lymph node dissection. The sentinel lymph node and 11 of 16 lymph nodes were positive for tumor. Estrogen receptors and progesterone receptors were both positive. Further staging work-up was negative for distant metastasis. Her final staging was stage IIB. Her prescribed chemotherapy regimen is 6 cycles of CAF after a single-lumen central line was placed.

1. M.D. asks you to help her understand how big her tumor was.

2. Describe the biopsy technique used for this diagnosis.

3. Discuss the implications of a positive sentinel node.

4. Using the TNM staging system, what would her classification be?

5. What is the significance of her hormone receptor status?

6. Surgical intervention is called the primary treatment for breast cancer. Follow-up (F/U) chemotherapy is called what kind of therapy?

7. List the chemotherapy drugs used for her treatment. List any side effects and special considerations associated with the use of these drugs.

8. Calculate M.D.'s body surface area (m^2). Her height is 5'7", and her weight is 155 pounds.

9. Calculate the dose of her doxorubicin at 75 mg/m^2.

CASE STUDY PROGRESS

M.D. has now received 3 cycles of combination chemotherapy for her breast cancer. Her last treatment with doxorubicin, cyclophosphamide, and 5-fluorouracil was approximately 12 days ago. She came to the emergency department (ED) with a 2-day history of fever, chills, and shortness of breath (SOB). On arrival, she is disoriented and agitated. Vital signs (VS) are 86/43, 119, 28, 39.8°C, Sao$_2$ 85% on room air. Laboratory data include WBC 1.2 thou/cmm, Hct 24.9%, Hgb 8.7 g/dl, platelets 125 thou/cmm. Differential WBC count shows 37% granulocytes, 60% lymphocytes, 3% monocytes. Chem 14 is within normal limits (WNL), with the exception of BUN 28 mg/dl, creatinine 1.6 mg/dl, and lactic acid 2.4 mg/dl. Chest x-ray (CXR) demonstrates diffuse infiltrates in the left lower lung.

10. M.D.'s AGC is 444/cmm. What is the significance of an AGC of 444/cmm?

11. What are the probable causes of the abnormal laboratory findings listed above?

�֎ **12.** What is the single most important nursing intervention for a patient with an AGC less than 500/cmm?

13. What is the significance of the lactic acid level?

CASE STUDY PROGRESS

M.D.'s oxygen requirements significantly increase. She is admitted into the ICU and requires endotracheal intubation.

14. Differentiate among sepsis, severe sepsis, and septic shock.

CASE STUDY PROGRESS

M.D. spends 3 days in the ICU receiving antibiotics and respiratory support. She is able to be extubated and returns to the oncology unit, where she remains for a few more days before being discharged home.

Case Study **94**

Scenario

C.P. is a 71-year-old married farmer, with a past medical history (PMH) of hernia surgery in 1965 and prostate surgery in 1992 for benign prostatic hyperplasia (BPH). C.P. does not drink, but he has smoked for 40 years; the past 3 years he has smoked 2 to 3 packs per day (PPD). He has no known drug allergies (NKDA). Six months ago C.P. visited the local rural health clinic with complaints of (C/O) progressive cough and chest congestion. Despite a week of antibiotic therapy, C.P. continued to worsen; he experienced progressive dyspnea and productive cough, and he began to have night sweats. C.P. refuses to be admitted to the hospital ("There's no one to look after the cows") but agrees to go for a chest x-ray (CXR). The radiologist reads C.P.'s CXR as left hilar lung mass, probable lung cancer. C.P. is scheduled for a diagnostic fiberoptic bronchoscopy with endobronchial lung biopsy as an outpatient to confirm the diagnosis.

1. What is fiberoptic bronchoscopy, and what information will fiberoptic bronchoscopy with endobronchial lung biopsy provide?

2. As the nurse who works with the pulmonologist, it is your responsibility to prepare C.P. for the fiberoptic bronchoscopy procedure. What would you include in your teaching plan?

3. What is your responsibility during and immediately after the bronchoscopy?

4. C.P. tolerates the procedure well. He returns to the office in 4 days to learn the results of his test. The pulmonologist tells C.P. and his wife that he has poorly differentiated oat cell lung cancer and explains that it is a very fast–growing cancer with a poor prognosis. This kind of lung cancer is directly related to (R/T) C.P.'s history of smoking. What is your role at this time?

5. What does poorly differentiated mean?

CASE STUDY PROGRESS
C.P. is scheduled to begin combination chemotherapy with cisplatin (Platinol) and etoposide (VePesid). He plans to continue to work the farm as long as possible; his brother-in-law has promised to help him.

6. How would you explain combination chemotherapy and how it works to C.P. and his wife?

7. C.P.'s wife tells you she's heard that chemotherapy makes you really sick. How would you explain chemotherapy side effects?

8. What are the most common side effects of cisplatin and etoposide?

9. Based on your knowledge of the most common side effects, list at least seven interventions that should be incorporated into C.P.'s care plan.

10. C.P. needs to have a working understanding of how to balance his treatment with his work. You sit down with C.P. to plan a daily work, activity, rest schedule to accommodate his treatments and side effects. List at least four concepts you would emphasize.

11. C.P. receives cisplatin 60 mg in 100 ml normal saline (NS) IV over 1 to 2 hours daily, the first 3 days of each month for 6 months; and etoposide 200 mg in 250 ml NS IV over 1 to 2 hours daily, the first 3 days of each month for 6 months. What is the nadir for each drug, and what implications does the nadir have for C.P.?

CASE STUDY PROGRESS

A month later, when C.P. returns for his second round of chemotherapy, he complains of shortness of breath (SOB), chest tightness, and palpitations. He looks exhausted. ECG and CXR reveal atrial fibrillation (A-fib) and left lower lobe (LLL) pneumonia with pleural effusion. C.P. is admitted to the hospital with the following laboratory values: WBC 2.5 thou/cmm, RBC 4.9 mill/cmm, Hgb 12.7 g/dl, Hct 37.6%, platelets 152 thou/cmm, Na 131 mmol/L, K 4.2 mmol/L, Cl 90 mmol/L, CO_2 24 mEq/L, BUN 13 mg/dl, creatinine 0.8 mg/dl, glucose 105 mg/dl.

12. What do these lab values indicate?

13. The pulmonologist performs a thoracentesis and prescribes cefotaxime 1 g IV q8h and erythromycin 500 mg IV q6h. What factor in C.P.'s background will complicate his diagnosis of pneumonia?

14. C.P.'s condition continues to deteriorate. He tells you he doesn't want to live like this, but the physician wants to continue with aggressive therapy. Discuss the pros and cons of continued therapy and what role you can play in helping him.

CASE STUDY PROGRESS

C.P. refuses the second round of chemotherapy and is discharged to home. He receives no further treatment and dies 2 weeks later—on his own terms.

Case Study **95**

Name _____ Class/Group _____ Date _____
Group Members _____
INSTRUCTIONS All questions apply to this case study. Your responses should be brief and to the point. When asked to provide several answers, list them in order of priority or significance. Do not assume information that is not provided. Please print or write clearly. If your response is not legible, it will be marked as ? and you will need to rewrite it.

Scenario

H.J. is a 46-year-old man diagnosed with Burkitt's lymphoma 4 months ago. He has received 3 of 6 chemotherapy courses and is seen today at his physician's office with a complaint of (C/O) malaise and fever. He is found to have splenomegaly on examination. In the office, his laboratory studies reveal WBC 51.9 thou/cmm, Hgb 8.3 g/dl, Hct 23.6%, platelets 21 thou/cmm. Differential shows neutrophils 66%, lymphocytes 16%, monocytes 15%, eosinophils 5%. He is admitted to the hospital with progressive disease.

On admission, further laboratory studies reveal Na 136 mmol/L, K 5.2 mmol/L, Cl 97 mmol/L, CO_2 28 mmol/L, glucose 98 mg/dl, BUN 24 mg/dl, creatinine 1.7 mg/dl, Ca 11.9 units/L, phosphorus 4.5 mg/dl, uric acid 23.7 mg/dl, total bilirubin 0.8 mg/dl, alkaline phosphatase 172 units/L, aspartate transaminase (AST) 254 units/L, alanine transaminase (ALT) 72 units/L, lactate dehydrogenase (LDH) 214 IU/L. CT of the abdomen shows a large spleen with metastatic disease in the liver, spleen, and pancreas; chest x-ray (CXR) demonstrates patchy infiltrates in bilateral lower lobes, R > L.

1. H.J. is diagnosed with acute tumor lysis syndrome. Briefly describe this syndrome.

2. Which of the above labs confirm this diagnosis?

3. List common signs and symptoms (S/S) of each metabolic abnormality associated with acute tumor lysis syndrome listed below.

4. The physician orders aggressive hydration, allopurinol, and chemotherapy to be started. He also ordered rasburicase, a new drug that decreases uric acid levels. How does this drug work?

5. Identify two additional complications or emergencies for which H.J. is at risk.

6. On hospital day 5, labs are as follows: WBC 1.4 thou/cmm, Hgb 8.3 g/dl, Hct 23.8%, platelets 10 thou/cmm, Na 138 mmol/L, K 4.8 mmol/L, Cl 109 mmol/L, CO_2 26 mmol/L, glucose 148 mg/dl, BUN 34 mg/dl, creatinine 1.0 mg/dl, Ca 7.3 units/L, total protein 5.4 g/dl, albumin 2.8 g/dl, phosphorus 3.8 mg/dl, uric acid less than 0.5 mg/dl, total bilirubin 1.0 mg/dl, alkaline phosphatase 96 units/L, AST 49 units/L, ALT 48 units/L, LDH 224 IU/L. Ordered chemotherapy has been completed. Comparing current laboratory data to those on admission, how has his condition changed?

7. H.J. required blood product support, including leukocyte-poor pheresed platelets and leukocyte-reduced packed RBCs (PRBCs). Acetaminophen and diphenhydramine (Benadryl) are ordered as premedication for transfusion. H.J. will be closely monitored for intravascular and extravascular hemolytic reactions; febrile, allergic, and hypervolemic reactions; transfusion-related acute lung injury (TRALI); and bacterial sepsis. Identify the S/S, usual cause, and treatment for each.

Case Study **96**

Scenario

R.M. is a 42-year-old woman with a history of stage IV ovarian carcinoma. She has previously been
treated surgically with an exploratory laparotomy that included a total abdominal hysterectomy (TAH),
an ileocecal resection and anastomosis, omentectomy, and peritoneal biopsies. Postoperative CA-125
level was 169 units/ml; currently it is 228 units/ml. She has received 3 courses of chemotherapy consisting of docetaxel and cisplatin. She is currently admitted with shortness of breath (SOB), complaints
of (C/O) nausea, and early satiety with recent weight loss of 10 pounds. Her abdomen is distended,
and her Sao$_2$ is 86% on room air.

1. What is the most common reason ovarian cancer is usually stage III or stage IV when
   initially diagnosed?

2. List three common presenting signs and symptoms of ovarian cancer.

3. Explain the significance of R.M.'s CA–125 levels.

4. R.M.'s chest x-ray (CXR) reveals bilateral pleural effusions. How do these relate to her
   underlying disease? How might they be treated?

5. Knowing the chemotherapeutic agents she has received, the nurse will closely monitor what laboratory data?

6. Identify five side effects of R.M's chemotherapeutic agents.

7. Surgical intervention at this time will include debulking of tumor and possible placement of a colostomy. Delineate four appropriate topics to be included in preoperative teaching.

8. R.M. is undergoing a palliative surgical intervention. How would the nurse explain this to the patient and family?

9. Family history analysis reveals a strong positive occurrence of breast and ovarian cancer in R.M.'s family. Her mother died of breast cancer at the age of 56, and a maternal aunt died of ovarian cancer at the age of 59. At the onset of her illness, the physician suggested the possibility of testing for the presence of the *BRAC1* and *BRAC2* genes. Describe the meaning of this test.

10. Discuss pros and cons of genetic testing for cancer.

11. R.M. tested positive for the *BRAC2* gene. What implications might this result have for her children?

Case Study **97**

Name _____ Class/Group _____ Date _____
Group Members _____

INSTRUCTIONS All questions apply to this case study. Your responses should be brief and to the point. When asked
to provide several answers, list them in order of priority or significance. Do not assume information that is not provided.
Please print or write clearly. If your response is not legible, it will be marked as ? and you will need to rewrite it.

Scenario

V.M. is a 39-year-old African-American man who has sickle cell disease (SCD), sometimes called
sickle cell anemia, marked by frequent episodes of severe pain. His anemia has been managed with
multiple transfusions, and he shows signs of chronic renal failure. He is a nonsmoker and nondrinker
and is on Social Security disability. His regular medications are pentoxifylline (Trental), oxycodone-
acetaminophen, and folic acid. In the hematology clinic this morning, V.M.'s hemoglobin (Hgb)
measures 6.7 g/dl. He received 2 units packed RBCs (PRBCs) over 3 hours and then went home. He
developed dyspnea and shortness of breath (SOB) approximately 1 to 1½ hours later, and his wife
called 911. The emergency medical system (EMS) crew initiated oxygen (O_2) and transported V.M. to
the emergency department (ED).

1. What is SCD, and how is it related to race?

2. The stiff, sickled RBCs tend to cause vascular occlusions with subsequent local infarction.
As a rule, the spleen suffers so many vasoocclusive/infarction episodes that it is greatly
reduced in size and is rendered nonfunctional by the time the individual is 6 years of age.
What are the implications of having a nonfunctioning spleen?

3. Identify two mechanisms that contribute to anemia in patients with SCD.

4. When V.M. arrives at the ED, the physician asks him if he is in pain and if he needs a narcotic. V.M. answers no to both questions. Why did the physician ask these two questions?

5. V.M.'s arterial blood gases (ABGs) on 9 L O_2 by simple face mask show Pao_2 (partial pressure of oxygen in arterial blood) 74 mm Hg. Is V.M. being adequately oxygenated?

6. V.M. complains of (C/O) being SOB. Do you believe his low Hgb level is responsible for his complaints?

CASE STUDY PROGRESS

You perform a quick assessment and note a systolic murmur and crackles in V.M.'s bases bilaterally. Vital signs (VS) are 176/102, 94, 28, 97°F (oral). Acting according to the standing orders for your institution, you start an IV and draw blood for CBC with differential, basic metabolic panel (BMP), calcium, and phosphorus and send it for analysis.

7. Your assessment findings are consistent with fluid overload. What four findings led you to that conclusion?

8. What action would you expect the physician to take next, and why?

CASE STUDY PROGRESS

The lab values return: Na 137 mmol/L, K 4.9 mmol/L, Cl 110 mmol/L, CO_2 16 mmol/L, BUN 27 mg/dl, creatinine 2.7 mg/dl, Ca 8.2 mg/dl, phosphate 4.7 mg/dl, WBC 4.3 thou/cmm, Hgb 7.8 g/dl, Hct 20.9%, platelets 208 thou/cmm.

9. What is the significance of the lab results, and why?

CASE STUDY PROGRESS

The physician prescribes furosemide (Lasix) 20 mg IV push (IVP) now, methylprednisolone (Solu-Medrol) 125 mg IVP, and ceftriaxone (Rocephin) 1 g IV piggyback (IVPB) after the furosemide.

10. What is the significance of each of these drugs?

11. Why is it difficult to crossmatch blood to transfuse V.M.? What precautions should be taken with each unit of blood?

CASE STUDY PROGRESS

As V.M.'s SOB is relieved, he shakes the physician's hand and thanks him for asking about the presence of pain and the need for pain medication. V.M. states, "One of my biggest fears is that I'll come in here in crisis and the doctor won't treat my pain aggressively enough. I don't want to be labeled as a drug seeker or an emergency room abuser."

12. Why would V.M. be concerned about obtaining adequate pain control in the ED?

CASE STUDY PROGRESS

V.M. voids 1900 ml within 2 hours of the furosemide administration. On repeat assessment, the systolic murmur is audible, but all lung fields are clear. Repeat VS are 160/94, 82, 20, 98° F (oral). V.M. is discharged on his previous medications.

13. What issues would you address with V.M. before discharge?

Case Study **98**

Scenario

C.O. is a 43-year-old woman who noted a nonpruritic nodular rash on her neck and chest approximately 6 weeks ago. Other symptoms she noted were polyarticular joint pain and back pain. The rash became generalized, spreading to her head, abdomen, and arms. She experienced 3 episodes of epistaxis in 1 day about 2 weeks ago. Over the past week, her gums have become swollen and tender. Because of the progression of symptoms and increasing fatigue, she sought medical attention. Lab work was performed, and C.O. was referred to a hematologist.

The CBC revealed WBC 39 thou/cmm, Hgb 10.4 g/dl, Hct 28.7%, platelets 49 thou/cmm. The WBC differential was monocytes 64%, lymphocytes 15%, neutrophils 4%, blasts 17%. Chemistry studies came back Na 139 mmol/L, K 3.2 mmol/L, Cl 100 mmol/L, CO_2 32 mmol/L, BUN 14 mg/dl, creatinine 1.0 mg/dl, glucose 140 mg/dl, lactate dehydrogenase (LDH) 1850 units/L, uric acid 6.1 mg/dl. The chest x-ray (CXR) showed normal lung expansion, heart size normal, and no lymphadenopathy. Skin biopsy showed cutaneous leukemic infiltrates, and a bone marrow biopsy showed moderately hypercellular marrow and collections of monoblasts. The final diagnosis was acute myeloblastic leukemia.

C.O. is admitted to the hematology/oncology unit of a teaching hospital. She is to receive cytarabine (Ara-C, Cytosar) 100 mg/m²/day as continuous infusion for 7 days and idarubicin 12 mg/m²/day IV push (IVP) for 3 days. She is scheduled in angiography for placement of a triple-lumen subclavian Hickman catheter before beginning her therapy. A lumbar puncture for routine studies and cytology will also be performed.

1. Interpret the CBC. What does the presence of blasts in the differential mean?

2. What is the purpose of a bone marrow biopsy?

3. Considering all the admission data listed above, what potential problem will the nurse be alert for after the patient returns to the unit following insertion of the catheter?

4. What assessments are essential for the nurse to make regarding the central catheter throughout the hospitalization?

5. What are the side effects related to the following chemotherapeutic agents: cytarabine and idarubicin? Identify five nursing interventions related to the side effects of each chemotherapeutic agent.

CASE STUDY PROGRESS

On the fifth day of continuous infusion of cytarabine, C.O. develops a fever of 38.6°C. Her vital signs (VS) are 110/54, 115, 26. The nurse notifies the intern on duty, who evaluates the patient and writes the following orders: blood cultures ×2 sites; Tylenol suppository 650 mg PR q4-6h prn; Primaxin 500 mg IVPB q8h; notify MD of T > 38.5°C.

6. Do these orders seem appropriate for this patient? Explain.

7. Daily labs are drawn. On the last day of the continuous chemotherapy, C.O.'s CBC showed WBC 1.2 thou/cmm, Hgb 6.8 g/dl, Hct 21.3%, platelets 17 thou/cmm, differential bands 0%, neutrophils 5%, monocytes 25%, lymphocytes 65%, blasts 5%. What does this count indicate about her immune system?

8. Considering the above mentioned data, what blood products will most likely be ordered for C.O.?

9. On day 14 after completion of her therapy, a bone marrow biopsy shows the patient is in complete remission. With continued blood product support and antibiotic coverage, her marrow recovers and she is discharged from the hospital. HLA (human lymphocyte antigen) typing has been performed on all siblings. Her oldest brother is a perfect HLA match and has agreed to donate bone marrow or stem cells. C.O. is to be readmitted to the bone marrow transplant unit within the next few weeks. What does "complete remission" mean for C.O.?

10. What type of bone marrow transplant will she have? Briefly describe the transplant process.

11. On day 17 after the transplant, she develops severe nausea and vomiting (N/V) in addition to diarrhea of more than 1200 cc/24 hr. She is made NPO. Graft–versus–host disease of the gut is suspected. Describe graft–versus–host disease. How would the nurse explain this to the patient and her family? Is there a potentially positive result of this complication? Explain your answer.

12. Identify four problems, then develop interventions and expected outcomes, for a patient undergoing a bone marrow transplant.

chapter

10

Pediatric Disorders

Case Study **99**

Name _____ Class/Group _____ Date _____
Group Members _____
INSTRUCTIONS All questions apply to this case study. Your responses should be brief and to the point. When asked
to provide several answers, list them in order of priority or significance. Do not assume information that is not provided.
Please print or write clearly. If your response is not legible, it will be marked as ? and you will need to rewrite it.

Scenario

A.P. is an 8-year-old who is sent to the nurse's office because she has had a several-day history of
scratching her head so badly that she complains that her "head hurts." You complete a general examination of A.P.'s head and notice that she has red, irritated areas with several scratch marks; a few
open sores; and sesame seed–sized, silvery white and yellow nodules (bugs) that are adhered to many
of her hair shafts. You determine that A.P. has pediculosis capitis.

1. What is pediculosis capitis?

2. What will be your next steps in A.P.'s care?

3. What should be included in the educational plans for A.P. and her parents?

4. Why would head lice occur in school-aged children?

5. What possible complications can occur as a result of failing to treat head lice?

6. What should your nursing actions include regarding A.P.'s classmates?

Case Study **100**

Name _____ Class/Group _____ Date _____
Group Members _____

INSTRUCTIONS All questions apply to this case study. Your responses should be brief and to the point. When asked to provide several answers, list them in order of priority or significance. Do not assume information that is not provided. Please print or write clearly. If your response is not legible, it will be marked as ? and you will need to rewrite it.

Scenario

Z.O. is a 3-year-old boy with no significant medical history. He is brought into the emergency department (ED) by the emergency medical technicians (EMTs) after experiencing a seizure lasting 3 minutes. His parents report no previous history that may contribute to the seizure, although they have noticed that he has been irritable, has had a poor appetite, and has been more clumsy than usual over the past 2 to 3 weeks. CT scan of the brain shows a 1-cm mass in the posterior fossa region of the brain. The physician suspects a cerebellar astrocytoma.

1. What are the most common presenting symptoms of a brain tumor?

2. Primary treatment for this child is surgical resection followed by external beam radiation. Describe some of the criteria the neurosurgeon will use to determine the appropriateness of surgery in this case.

3. Why are many chemotherapeutic drugs ineffective in the treatment of lesions in the central nervous system (CNS)?

4. Discuss some of the issues Z.O.'s parents will experience during the immediate postoperative period.

5. Z.O. has a 5-year-old sister. She has been afraid of visiting at the hospital. Delineate four strategies to help siblings cope with the illness of a sibling.

6. Postoperatively, Z.O. completed a 6-week course of radiotherapy. Now, 4 months later, he is experiencing new symptoms, including behavior changes and regression in speech and mobility. His tumor has recurred. The physician suggests hospice care to Z.O.'s parents. List some of the goals of hospice care for this patient and family.

CASE STUDY PROGRESS

Z.O. dies at home just before his fourth birthday. To deal with their grief, the family becomes involved with the Candlelighter's Childhood Cancer Foundation *(http://www.candlelighters.org)*. Access this website and review some of the services available to children with cancer and their families.

Case Study **101**

Scenario

S.G. is a 13-month-old girl who is scheduled for repair of her cleft palate. Her mother brings her to the same-day surgery unit at 0630 on the morning of her scheduled surgery. Your preoperative assessment findings include vital signs (VS) 98/68, 136, 36 and slightly labored, 39.5°C (tympanic); breath sounds diminished throughout with congestion noted bilaterally; Sao$_2$ 90%; color pale pink; weight 9.5 kg.

1. Which of these assessment findings are of concern and why?

2. Based on these findings, what will most likely occur regarding surgery?

3. The plastic surgeon cancels S.G.'s surgery. What information and support should you give to Mrs. G. at this time?

4. S.G.'s weight and height are plotted on a growth chart. She is found to fall below the 5th percentile for both. What additional information should you gather from Mrs. G.?

5. What is the significance of S.G.'s height and weight in terms of her chances of recovering from surgery and future growth and development?

6. Identify the members of the interdisciplinary health care team and the roles and responsibilities each will have while working with S.G. and her parents. What is your rationale for including each member?

Case Study **102**

Scenario

S.B. is the only child of Mr. and Mrs. B. The family has been living out of their car for the past 2 months; Mr. B. lost his job 2 weeks after S.B.'s birth and looks for work every day. Mrs. B. takes advantage of the good weather and spends most of the day playing with S.B. in the park. As the triage nurse in the emergency department (ED), you ask why they have brought S.B. to the hospital. Mrs. B. states that S.B. breast fed well for the first couple of weeks, but since then "throws up all the time like he's forcing all his feedings out. He looks skinny and sick, and he cries and is fussy all the time."

1. What additional information will you need to obtain from Mr. and Mrs. B.?

2. What would you include in your physical assessment of S.B.?

3. The emergency physician orders lab work and x-rays. What labs would you expect to be ordered, and what results would you expect to find knowing that S.B. has been vomiting frequently and that he may be diagnosed with dehydration and metabolic alkalosis?

4. What is the underlying cause for S.B.'s diagnosis of metabolic alkalosis?

5. What physical assessment findings occur with metabolic alkalosis?

6. What additional assessment findings might reflect the consequences of frequent vomiting in the infant?

CASE STUDY PROGRESS

S.B. is diagnosed with pyloric stenosis, admitted to the pediatric unit, and scheduled for surgery. S.B.'s parents are worried because they have no insurance and "don't want anything bad to happen to our baby."

7. What are your responsibilities as you admit S.B. and get him ready for surgery?

8. What are the implications of the family's homelessness, financial situation, and lack of insurance?

Case Study **103**

Scenario

K.B. is a 16-year-old who fell while skiing. She was transported down the hill by the ski patrol after being stabilized and then was flown to the hospital. She has a fractured right femur and humerus. She is admitted to your unit after an open reduction and internal fixation (ORIF) of the femur fracture and casting of her leg and arm.

1. What information should you receive from the postanesthesia care unit (PACU) nurse?

2. How will you use this information in planning your immediate assessment and care of K.B.?

❀ **3.** Prioritize the following orders from the most to the least important, and be prepared to explain the priorities you assigned.

____ A. Vital signs (VS) per routine

____ B. Neurologic checks q2h

____ C. Turn, cough, and deep breathe (TCDB) and incentive spirometer (IS) q2h while awake

____ D. Ice and elevate right lower extremity and right upper extremity

____ E. Circulation, movement, sensation (CMS) checks q1h

____ F. NPO

____ G. IV fluids D_5.45NS at 100 ml/hr

____ H. Morphine sulfate 1 to 2 mg IV q4-6h prn

____ I. Cefazolin (Ancef) 880 mg IV q6h

CASE STUDY PROGRESS

K.B. has been on the unit for approximately 6 hours. You identify the following changes in your assessment data: K.B. is difficult to arouse, but when awake is able to identify who and where she is; PERRLA (*Pupils Equal, Round, Reactive to Light and Accommodation*) is 1+ with slower reaction time than earlier; color is pale, pink; skin is cool and clammy; heart rate is 126 beats/min, respiratory rate is 28 breaths/min, temperature (oral) is 39°C; Sao$_2$ is 90%. You find that neurovascular checks of the affected extremities are unchanged.

❋ 4. What should your immediate nursing interventions include?

5. What information should you report to the orthopedic surgeon, and what is your rationale for doing so?

6. K.B.'s Glasgow Coma Scale begins to decline. What are possible reasons for changes in her neurologic status?

CASE STUDY PROGRESS

K.B. spent 12 hours in the pediatric ICU being monitored for changes in her neurologic status. Her primary health care provider (PCP) determined she was stable and had her transferred to the pediatric unit. It is now 24 hours postop. K.B. suddenly begins to complain of extreme pain in her lower right leg. Your assessment finds right foot cool, pale, with an absent pedal pulse and decreased mobility.

✳ 7. What is the most likely cause of these changes, and what should your immediate response be?

8. K.B.'s cast is split and her foot pulses are restored. K.B. and her parents are extremely anxious. What education and support should be provided to K.B. and her parents?

Case Study **104**

Scenario

J.R., a 13-year-old with cystic fibrosis, is being seen in the outpatient clinic for a biannual evaluation. J.R. lives at home with his parents and 7-year-old sister, C.R., who also has cystic fibrosis. J.R. reports that he "doesn't feel good," explaining that he has missed the last week of school, doesn't have any energy, is coughing more, and is having "a hard time breathing."

1. What additional data should be obtained from J.R. and his parents?

CASE STUDY PROGRESS

J.R. is admitted to the hospital for a pulmonary "clean-out." Your assessment includes the following: color pale pink with bluish tinged nail beds; respiratory rate 28 breaths/min and somewhat labored; temperature 38.8°C (oral); Sao$_2$ 88%; rhonchi noted throughout; thorax has a barrel chest appearance; appears thin, weighs 30 kg.

2. Why is J.R. at risk for developing pulmonary infections?

3. What are the common microorganisms that cause respiratory infections in children with cystic fibrosis?

4. J.R.'s physician orders ceftazidime 2 g IV q8h, gentamicin 160 mg IV q8h, and vancomycin 650 mg IV q8h. What should you do before administering these drugs?

CASE STUDY PROGRESS

The following are recommended dosages:

Ceftazidime

Infants and children: 90 to 150 mg/kg q8h
Adults: 1 to 2 g q8h; maximum of 2 g q6h
Minimum: 90 × 30 = 2700 mg/day = 900 mg/dose
Maximum: 150 × 30 = 4500 mg/day = 1500 mg/dose

Gentamicin

Infants and children: 7.5 to 10.5 mg/kg q8h
Minimum: 7.5 mg × 30 = 225 mg/day = 75 mg/dose
Maximum: 10.5 × 30 = 315 mg/day = 105 mg/dose

Vancomycin

Infants and children: 40 mg/kg q8h
Adults: 500 mg q6h
Dosage: 40 × 30 = 1200 mg/day = 400 mg/dose

5. Are the dosages prescribed for J.R. within a safe range? What factor will affect the selection of antibiotics and their dosages?

6. What are other commonly prescribed medications that children with cystic fibrosis take on a daily basis? Why are these important?

7. J.R.'s weight is below the 5th percentile. He has been on a high-calorie, high-protein diet at home; however, he reports that he hasn't been hungry and really hasn't been eating much. What is the link between malnutrition and cystic fibrosis?

8. What clinical sign assists in determining the effective dosage of pancreatic enzymes?

9. J.R. will be spending 14 to 21 days in the hospital for his pulmonary clean-out. How will this hospitalization affect J.R.'s normal development? How can you foster his development while he is hospitalized?

10. Identify four long-term complications associated with cystic fibrosis.

11. Is lung transplantation successful for children with cystic fibrosis?

Case Study **105**

Scenario

J.H. is a 2-week-old infant brought to the emergency department (ED) by his mother, who speaks little English. Her husband is at work. She is young and appears frightened and anxious. Through a translator, Mrs. H. reports that J.H. has not been eating, sleeps all the time, and is "not normal."

1. What should your assessment include?

2. What are some of the obstacles you need to consider, recognizing that Mrs. H. does not speak or understand English well?

CASE STUDY PROGRESS

The ED physician orders the following lab work: CBC with differential; blood culture; complete metabolic panel (CMP); urinalysis (UA); and cerebrospinal fluid (CSF) for culture, glucose, protein, cell count (following a lumbar puncture). J.H. is admitted to the medical unit with a diagnosis of rule out (R/O) sepsis and meningitis.

3. What lab values would you anticipate being above normal and why?

✤ **4.** What would your priority nursing care include after his admission assessment?

✤ **5.** J.H. is diagnosed with *Escherichia coli* meningitis. His medical care plan will include 14 to 21 days of antibiotic therapy. In addition to monitoring his neurologic status, identify three things you will include in your care plan for J.H.

6. How will you involve his parents?

7. What is the impact of hospitalization on J.H.'s growth and development?

8. J.H. is being discharged after 3 weeks of IV antibiotic therapy. What educational topics will be important to discuss with J.H.'s parents when he is discharged?

Case Study **106**

Name _____ Class/Group _____ Date _____
Group Members _____
INSTRUCTIONS All questions apply to this case study. Your responses should be brief and to the point. When asked to provide several answers, list them in order of priority or significance. Do not assume information that is not provided. Please print or write clearly. If your response is not legible, it will be marked as ? and you will need to rewrite it.

Scenario

L.S. is a 7-year-old who is being directly admitted to your unit from his pediatrician's office. His mother has brought him directly to the unit without stopping to admit him. She immediately tells you that she is a single parent and has 2 other children at home with a babysitter. Your assessment finds L.S. alert, oriented, and extremely anxious. His color is pale, and his nail beds are dusky and cool to the touch; other findings are heart rate 136 beats/min, respiratory rate 36 breaths/min regular and even, oral temperature 37.3°C, Sao_2 92%, breath sounds decreased in lower lobes bilaterally and congested with inspiratory and expiratory wheezes, prolonged expirations.

1. As you ask Mrs. S. questions, you note that L.S.'s respiratory rate is increasing; he is sitting on the side of the bed, leaning slightly forward, and is having difficulty breathing. What should your immediate nursing care include?

2. Prioritize the following orders from the most to the least important, and be prepared to explain your order of priority.
_____ A. Vital signs (VS) q2h
_____ B. Cardiac and respiratory monitor
_____ C. Continuous pulse oximeter
_____ D. IV fluids, D_5.45NS at 78 ml/hr
_____ E. Chest x-ray (CXR) STAT
_____ F. Arterial blood gases (ABGs) STAT
_____ G. Give a loading dose of aminophylline 240 mg IV over 30 minutes, then maintain an aminophylline drip of 0.9 mg/kg/hr
_____ H. Methylprednisolone (Solu-Medrol) 40 mg IV q6h
_____ I. Albuterol 2.5 mg inhaled now and q3-4h prn

3. Identify the nursing responsibilities associated with giving aminophylline and albuterol.

✻ **4.** Asthma education is ordered for L.S. and his mother. You call her to arrange a schedule. You find out that the phone number she has provided is no longer in service. What should be your next nursing action?

CASE STUDY PROGRESS

Mrs. S. arrives to visit L.S. later that day, and you begin to discuss the education plan and to arrange when Mrs. S. can participate. You learn that Mrs. S. works 12 hours a day, the family is not covered by insurance, and she is worried about how she will pay for the hospitalization and medications for her son.

✻ **5.** What will be your next step, and how might this information influence your discharge planning?

6. L.S. tells you that he loves to play basketball and football and asks you if he can still do these activities. How should you respond?

7. What information should be included in your discharge teaching regarding how to prevent acute asthmatic episodes and to manage symptoms of exacerbation of asthma?

More information can be found at:

American Lung Association: *http://www.lungusa.org*

Asthma and Allergy Foundation of America: *http://www.aafa.org*

Asthmacontrol.com: *http://www.asthmacontrol.com*

GinaAsthma.com: *http://www.ginaasthma.com*

National Heart, Lung, and Blood Institute: *http://www.nhlbi.nih.gov*

Case Study **107**

Name _____ Class/Group_____ Date _____
Group Members _____
INSTRUCTIONS All questions apply to this case study. Your responses should be brief and to the point. When asked
to provide several answers, list them in order of priority or significance. Do not assume information that is not provided.
Please print or write clearly. If your response is not legible, it will be marked as ? and you will need to rewrite it.

Scenario

E.M., a 5-month-old girl, has been admitted for respiratory distress, hypoxia, and fever. Her viral respiratory panel shows that she has respiratory syncytial virus (RSV). In the emergency department (ED), her Sao_2 was 78% on room air, and she was placed on 1.5 L oxygen (O_2). On admission to the floor, the patient is fussy and difficult to console. Vital signs (VS) are 130/72, 188, 83, 38.4°C (rectal), and Sao_2 94% on 1.5 L O_2.

1. Based on the patient's diagnosis, what else would be important to assess?

2. You provide nasopharyngeal suction for the patient and obtain a moderate amount of thick secretions. After allowing the patient to recover, you reassess the patient's respiratory status. The respiratory rate and retractions have not changed significantly. The breath sounds are less coarse, but they are diminished in the bases. The Sao_2 is now 90% on 1.5 L O_2. E.M.'s mother asks if she can feed the patient, since she has not eaten much for the past 3 days. You tell her that with the patient's respiratory rate greater than 65 breaths/min, she should not be fed. What is the rationale for holding feeds?

3. When you call the primary care provider (PCP), you are given orders for an albuterol nebulizer trial, IV bolus, and acetaminophen for the fever. What is the rationale for the albuterol trial?

4. How will an IV bolus improve E.M.'s respiratory status?

�֎ **5.** Prioritize the following doctor's orders, and give your rationale.

  ____ A. Acetaminophen 60 mg PO for fever

  ____ B. D$_5$LR 80 ml IV bolus

  ____ C. Albuterol 2.5 mg inhaled

6. Mrs. M. asks why the physician is not prescribing antibiotics. What would you tell her?

CASE STUDY PROGRESS

After the albuterol treatment, the respiratory rate is 23 breaths/min, and the retractions have increased. The Sao$_2$ is 89% on 2 L of O$_2$. E.M. is pale and listless and does not cry when the IV is placed.

7. Why is the respiratory rate significantly lower even though other signs of respiratory distress have increased?

CASE STUDY PROGRESS

The PCP orders a portable chest x-ray (CXR) and capillary blood gas (CBG). The CXR is consistent with bronchiolitis with atelectasis. The CBG was pH 7.31, Pco$_2$ 72 mm Hg, HCO$_2$ 29 mEq/L.

8. Is the patient in acidosis or alkalosis? Respiratory or metabolic? Explain the results based on the patient's condition.

CASE STUDY PROGRESS

E.M. is placed on a continuous positive airway pressure (CPAP) machine. You know from experience that patients are usually on CPAP for a couple days before they are ready to be taken off and continue to improve until they are ready for discharge. However, Mrs. M. is very distressed and asks you, "When is my baby going to die?" When you tell her that the patient is very sick but not dying, she says emphatically, "You can tell me. When is my baby going to die?"

9. What would you say to her?

Case Study 108

Name _____ Class/Group _____ Date _____

Group Members _____

INSTRUCTIONS All questions apply to this case study. Your responses should be brief and to the point. When asked to provide several answers, list them in order of priority or significance. Do not assume information that is not provided. Please print or write clearly. If your response is not legible, it will be marked as ? and you will need to rewrite it.

Scenario

You admit L.M., a 2-month-old girl with a history of hydrocephalus and ventriculoperitoneal (VP) shunt placement 1 month earlier. Her parents report that she has been more irritable than usual and for the past 3 days has had emesis 5 or 6 times every day.

1. What is the pathophysiology of hydrocephalus?

2. How does a VP shunt help patients with hydrocephalus?

CASE STUDY PROGRESS

L.M.'s vital signs (VS) are 111/70, 182, 55, 38.8°C, Sao$_2$ 95% on room air. Her head appears large, the fontanel is slightly bulging, and pupils are equal and reactive. The occipital frontal circumference (OFC) is 44 cm, and her mother tells you that is 2 cm more than when she measured yesterday. Baby L.M. is awake, irritable, and fussy throughout your assessment. She has emesis, although her father tells you that she has not eaten for 5 hours while they were in the emergency department (ED). Breath sounds are clear, pulses are 2+ and equal bilaterally, and capillary refill time is less than 2 sec.

3. Which of the vital signs and assessments are abnormal, and what are their possible causes?

4. In infants, why does the OFC increase when the pressure increases in the cranial vault?

5. The doctors order a CT scan and lumbar puncture with a cell count, culture, Gram stain, glucose, and protein run on the cerebrospinal fluid (CSF). What is the rationale for each procedure?

6. L.M. is taken to surgery to have an extraventricular drain (EVD) placed. What *categories* of medications might you expect the physicians to order postoperatively? Give the rationale for each category.

7. What should you teach the parents about the EVD?

8. Two days after the EVD is placed, L.M.'s father tells you that he is feeling discouraged because this is likely the first of many admission due to shunt malfunctions. He states that he talked to some parents of a child with hydrocephalus who was admitted 14 times by the time he was 2 years old. How would you respond to this father's feelings?

9. Later that day, Mrs. M. is changing L.M.'s diaper, and she tells you that she is worried because L.M. has started having diarrhea recently and it is getting worse. Based on the medications that the patient is getting, what is the most likely cause of the diarrhea? What is a possible concern you should consider, and what should your care plan include?

Case Study **109**

Name _____ Class/Group _____ Date _____
Group Members _____

INSTRUCTIONS All questions apply to this case study. Your responses should be brief and to the point. When asked to provide several answers, list them in order of priority or significance. Do not assume information that is not provided. Please print or write clearly. If your response is not legible, it will be marked as ? and you will need to rewrite it.

Scenario

The charge nurse tells you that you will be admitting a 1-hour-old girl, Baby Girl R., with a myelomeningocele that was discovered in utero. You know that the mother will still be at the local medical center recovering from her cesarean delivery.

1. What is the rationale for doing a cesarean delivery for babies with myelomeningocele?

CASE STUDY PROGRESS

The infant arrives accompanied by an aunt. The aunt tells you that the father will be coming later that day. While the aide is getting vital signs (VS), the aunt tells you that she has been trying to research myelomeningocele on the Internet, but she is still confused, especially about the difference between myelomeningocele and meningocele.

2. Using lay terms, what would you tell the aunt about the pathophysiology of myelomeningocele? What is the difference between myelomeningocele and meningocele?

CASE STUDY PROGRESS

Baby Girl R. is in an open warmer, and her VS are 67/33, 173, 52, 37.1°C (rectal), Sao$_2$ 95%. The fontanel is soft and flat; pupils are difficult to assess because the patient's eyes are closed, but they are 2 cm and react briskly. Baby Girl R. is sleepy, but she squirms and fusses when you check pupils. The sac in the sacral region is covered with moist gauze. Breath sounds are clear, bowel sounds are present, pulses are 2+, and capillary refill time is less than 3 sec. The infant has clubfeet, and she does not react at all when the pulse oximeter is placed on her right foot.

3. Which of the above assessment and monitoring data are abnormal for a 1-hour-old infant?

4. Explain the rationale for the following orders: Keep patient prone; start ampicillin and gentamicin; physical therapy (PT); open warmer; IV fluid; apply mud flap to sacral region below sac; place a Foley catheter; orthopedics consult; make NPO; keep sac gauze moist with normal saline (NS) (assess every hour).

CASE STUDY PROGRESS

The next day in report, you hear that Baby Girl R. did well overnight. She goes to surgery at 0815. Later, the postanesthesia care unit (PACU) nurse tells you that the patient is ready to come to your unit. When she arrives, you and your aide start putting on the monitors. Mr. R. is present, and he asks you to give the baby some pain medication. The open warmer starts alarming because the patient's skin temperature is reading 35.0° C. You look down at her to see if the temperature probe has fallen off. You see that it is still on, but you also notice that the suture from surgery is no longer intact. Then the oxygen (O_2) monitor reads 71% saturated with an accurate waveform, and the pulse oximeter probe is correctly placed on the patient.

5. Which of the issues should you address first? Give rationale.

CASE STUDY PROGRESS

Two days later, you are caring for Baby Girl R. at night. In report, you hear that the parents really want to hold their baby, but they have not yet because they are afraid of causing the suture to open again. They are currently at the bedside, and the infant is due for a feeding.

6. How can you help the parents become comfortable with holding their baby?

7. When you take the bottle in to the patient's room, you notice a growth chart next to the bed tracking the patient's occipital frontal circumference (OFC) that is measured at least once per shift. Why is the OFC monitored so closely on postoperative myelomeningocele patients?

Case Study **110**

Name _____ Class/Group _____ Date _____
Group Members _____

INSTRUCTIONS All questions apply to this case study. Your responses should be brief and to the point. When asked
to provide several answers, list them in order of priority or significance. Do not assume information that is not provided.
Please print or write clearly. If your response is not legible, it will be marked as ? and you will need to rewrite it.

Scenario

R.O. is a 12-year-old girl who lives with her family on a farm in a rural community. R.O. has 4 siblings
who have recently been ill with stomach pains, vomiting, diarrhea, and fever. They were seen by their
primary care provider (PCP) and diagnosed with viral gastroenteritis. A week later R.O. woke up at
0200 crying and telling her mother that her stomach "hurts really bad!" She had an elevated temperature of 37.9°C. R.O. began to vomit over the next few hours, so her parents took her to the local
emergency department (ED). R.O.'s vital signs (VS), CBC, complete metabolic panel (CMP) were normal,
so she was hydrated with IV fluids and discharged to home with instructions to call their PCP or to
return to the ED if she did not improve or worsened. Over the next 2 days, R.O.'s abdominal pain
localized to the right lower quadrant (RLQ), she refused to eat, and she had slight diarrhea. On the
third day she began to have more severe abdominal pain, increased vomiting, and fever that did not
respond to acetaminophen. R.O. returns to the ED. Her VS are 128/78, 130, 28, 39.5°C. Weight
is 42 kg, and height is 155 cm. R.O. is guarding her lower abdomen, prefers to lie on her side with
her legs flexed, and is crying. IV access is established, and morphine sulfate 2.0 mg IV is administered
for pain. An abdominal ultrasound (US) confirms a diagnosis of appendicitis. R.O.'s WBC is
25 thou/cmm.

1. Identify the clinical manifestations exhibited by R.O. that most clearly reflect the classic
   presentation of appendicitis.

2. Discuss why R.O.'s presenting clinical manifestations make diagnosis more difficult;
   identify two other possible diagnoses.

3. The abdominal US confirms that R.O. has appendicitis. What medical orders should you
   anticipate, and what is the rationale for them?

4. Mr. and Mrs. O. give informed consent, and R.O. assents to the surgery after the procedure is explained to her. Why is it important for R.O. to provide her assent for the procedure?

5. What should be included in the preoperative teaching for R.O. and her parents?

6. R.O. undergoes an appendectomy; the appendix has ruptured. The peritoneum is inflamed, and abscesses are seen near the colon and small intestine. R.O. is admitted to the surgical unit; she is NPO, has a nasogastric tube (NGT), Foley catheter, IV, abdominal dressing, and a Penrose drain. Identify five priority nursing considerations.

7. R.O. is 4 days postop. Assessment shows that R.O. is pale and listless; bowel sounds are absent; abdomen is distended and tender to the touch; the NGT is draining an increased amount of dark, greenish black fluid. Also, her lung sounds are moist bilaterally, her temperature has spiked to 40.2° C, and she rates her pain at 10/10 (she has been rating her pain from 5 to 7 on a scale of 1 to 10 for the past 2 days). R.O. has difficulty taking deep breaths because of the pain, which she says "hurts over my whole stomach." What should your priority nursing care include?

8. What information, if any, should you relate to her surgeon? What is your rationale for relating this information?

9. What lab work should you anticipate that the surgeon will order?

10. What should you consider as part of your nursing management of R.O.'s pain?

11. R.O. returns to surgery, where she has lysis of adhesions, removal of necrotic bowel, and drainage of an abscess. The surgeon has left her abdominal wound open and has ordered wound packing changes twice daily and abdominal irrigation with normal saline (NS). R.O. cries and becomes agitated when you go to perform the procedure. What should you consider in your approach to help R.O. cope with the procedure?

12. In anticipation of R.O.'s discharge, identify expected outcomes that must be achieved before her leaving the hospital. What will your discharge teaching include?

Case Study **111**

Name _____ Class/Group _____ Date _____
Group Members _____
INSTRUCTIONS All questions apply to this case study. Your responses should be brief and to the point. When asked
to provide several answers, list them in order of priority or significance. Do not assume information that is not provided.
Please print or write clearly. If your response is not legible, it will be marked as ? and you will need to rewrite it.

Scenario

T.M. is an 8-year-old with cerebral palsy who has been admitted to your unit following surgery for a
femoral osteotomy and tendon lengthening to stabilize hip joints and to help reduce spasticity. He is
admitted to your unit with a hip spica cast, an epidural for pain management, a Foley catheter, and a
gastrostomy tube (in place before the orthopedic surgery).

1. What are issues common to cerebral palsy that you should consider when planning and
   providing care to T.M.?

�֍ 2. What should be your top five priorities in providing nursing care to T.M.?

CASE STUDY PROGRESS

T.M. is 16 hours postop and is crying and extremely agitated, but is unable to communicate about what the problem is. His mother asks you to give him some diazepam.

3. What information should you gather from Mrs. M. to better understand her request for the medication?

4. What is the most likely reason Mrs. M. is requesting the diazepam?

✤ **5.** What should your next priority nursing intervention be?

6. It is 3 days since T.M. had surgery, and there is an order to remove his Foley catheter. What should your education and nursing plan include for T.M. and his mother?

7. You are discussing discharge plans with T.M. and his mother. What should be included in your discharge teaching?

chapter 11

Maternal and Obstetric Conditions

Case Study 112

Name _____ Class/Group _____ Date _____
Group Members _____
INSTRUCTIONS All questions apply to this case study. Your responses should be brief and to the point. When asked to provide several answers, list them in order of priority or significance. Do not assume information that is not provided. Please print or write clearly. If your response is not legible, it will be marked as ? and you will need to rewrite it.

Scenario

T.N. delivered a healthy male infant 2 hours ago. She had a midline episiotomy. This is her sixth pregnancy. She is para 4014. (Para indicates past history and does not list this delivery until later.) She had an epidural block for her labor and delivery. She is now admitted to the postpartum unit.

1. What is important to note in the initial assessment?

2. You find a boggy fundus during your assessment. What corrective measures can be instituted?

3. The patient complains of (C/O) pain and discomfort in her perineal area. How should you respond?

4. What patient teaching is vital for the nurse to do after delivery?

5. T.N. tells you she must go back to work in 6 weeks and isn't sure she can continue breast feeding. What options are available to her?

CASE STUDY PROGRESS

T.N. believes the AM and PM breast feeding schedule will work for her once she returns to work.

Case Study **113**

Name _____ Class/Group _____ Date _____
Group Members _____
INSTRUCTIONS All questions apply to this case study. Your responses should be brief and to the point. When asked to provide several answers, list them in order of priority or significance. Do not assume information that is not provided. Please print or write clearly. If your response is not legible, it will be marked as ? and you will need to rewrite it.

Scenario

P.M. comes to the obstetric (OB) clinic because she has missed 2 menstrual periods and thinks she may be pregnant. She states she is nauseated, especially in the AM, so she completed a home pregnancy test and it was positive. As the intake nurse in the clinic, you are responsible for gathering information before she sees the physician.

1. What are the two most important questions to ask to determine possible pregnancy?

2. She tells you she has never been pregnant. How would you record this information?

3. What additional information would be needed to complete the TPAL record?

4. It is important to complete the intake interview. What categories should you address with P.M.?

CASE STUDY PROGRESS

According to the clinic protocol, you obtain the following for her prenatal record: CBC, blood type, urine for urinalysis (UA) (protein, glucose, blood), vital signs (VS), height, and weight. Next, the physician or nurse-midwife does a physical examination, including a pelvic exam, and confirms P.M. is pregnant, the fetus is at approximately 6 weeks' gestation, and she has a gynecoid pelvis by measurement.

5. How would you calculate her due date?

6. What is the significance of a gynecoid pelvis?

CASE STUDY PROGRESS

Pregnancy is divided into 3 trimesters, each lasting about 3 months. Nursing interventions focus on monitoring the women and fetus for growth and development; detecting potential complications; and teaching P.M. about nutrition, how to deal with common discomforts of pregnancy, and activities of self-care.

7. A psychologic assessment is done to determine P.M.'s feelings and attitudes regarding her pregnancy. How do attitudes, beliefs, and feelings affect pregnancy?

8. As the nurse, you know that assessment and teaching are vital in the prenatal period to ensure a positive outcome. What information is important to include at every visit or at specific times during the pregnancy?

9. What are the "danger signs of pregnancy"?

10. Is a vaginal exam done at every visit? Why or why not?

CASE STUDY PROGRESS

An ultrasound (US) may be done at about 8 to 12 weeks' gestation to determine if the fetus is growing appropriately. The woman may be sent for a nonstress test after 36 weeks if risk factors dictate.

Case Study **114**

Name _____ Class/Group _____ Date _____
Group Members _____

INSTRUCTIONS All questions apply to this case study. Your responses should be brief and to the point. When asked to provide several answers, list them in order of priority or significance. Do not assume information that is not provided. Please print or write clearly. If your response is not legible, it will be marked as ? and you will need to rewrite it.

Scenario

You are the charge nurse working in labor and delivery at a local hospital. D.H. comes to the unit having contractions and feeling somewhat uncomfortable. You take her to the intake room to provide privacy, have her change into a gown, and ask her 3 initial questions to determine your next course of action, that is, whether to do a vaginal exam or to continue asking her more questions.

✺ **1.** What three initial questions should you ask and why?

2. D.H. has contractions 2 to 3 minutes apart and lasting 45 seconds. It is her third pregnancy (gravida 3, para 2002). Her bag of waters (BOW) is intact at this time. You determine it is appropriate to ask for further information before doing a vaginal exam. What information do you need?

3. What assessment should you make to gain further information from D.H.?

4. You check D.H.; she is 80% effaced and 4 cm dilated. The fetal heart rate (FHR) is 150 beats/min and regular. She is admitted to a labor and delivery room on the unit. What nursing measures should be done at this time?

5. Review the stages of labor. What stage is D.H. in?

6. It is vital to assess both mother and fetus throughout labor. What abnormalities should you look for?

7. You note a deceleration during a contraction. What should you do?

8. Decelerations occur in an early, variable, or late pattern. What is the significance of these patterns?

�֍ **9.** The remainder of the labor is uneventful; D.H. has an episiotomy to allow more room for the infant to emerge and delivers a male infant after 7 hours. What is involved in the immediate care of the newborn?

10. D.H. has her episiotomy repaired and the placenta delivered. What are the signs that the placenta has released from the uterine wall?

11. What assessments are important for D.H. following delivery?

Case Study **115**

Name _____ Class/Group _____ Date _____
Group Members _____

INSTRUCTIONS All questions apply to this case study. Your responses should be brief and to the point. When asked to provide several answers, list them in order of priority or significance. Do not assume information that is not provided. Please print or write clearly. If your response is not legible, it will be marked as ? and you will need to rewrite it.

Scenario

Baby H. is admitted to the transitional nursery, where the nurse will complete the physical assessment and observe for physiologic changes in the infant's transition from intrauterine to extrauterine life. The textbooks will tell you the infant goes through an initial phase of reactivity 30 to 60 minutes after birth, then a sleep phase for 4 to 6 hours, then a second period of reactivity. You will see variations of the timing in actual practice.

❋ **1.** What care is specific to the first period of reactivity?

2. The sleep phase and second reactive phase may occur in the nursery. Identify eight assessments or tasks that the nurse needs to do during the transitional care period.

3. Once the transitional care and documentation are completed, the infant is transferred to the normal newborn nursery. What ongoing care of newborn is this nurse responsible for?

4. What is the significance of the Coombs' test?

5. The baby is lethargic and not feeding well. What should your next action be?

6. Baby H.'s mother has decided to breast feed her infant. She asks for assistance. Identify six important points to include your teaching plan.

7. Baby H.'s mother asks you about cord care and circumcision care for her infant. What should you tell her?

8. You realize the baby needs follow-up (F/U) care after discharge. What should you teach the mother to help her understand the importance of regular visits?

9. You realize that Baby H.'s mother needs information about safety issues before being discharged. What should you teach her?

CASE STUDY PROGRESS

Baby H. is discharged to home with his parents.

Case Study **116**

Scenario

P.T. is a married 30-year-old gravida 4, para 1203 at 28 weeks' gestation. She arrives in the labor and delivery unit at a level 2 hospital complaining of low back pain and frequency of urination. She states that she feels occasional uterine cramping and believes that her membranes have not ruptured.

1. You are the charge nurse and admit P.T. Based on the information you have been given, identify the two most likely diagnoses for P.T.

2. What additional information do you need from P.T. to determine what you will do next?

3. What actions would you take to help identify her underlying problem before calling the health care provider?

4. What other problems might be going on with P.T. that you should consider?

CASE STUDY PROGRESS

P.T.'s history reveals that she had 1 preterm delivery 4 years ago at 31 weeks' gestation. The infant girl was in the neonatal intensive care unit (NICU) for 3 weeks and discharged without sequelae. The second preterm infant, a boy, was delivered 2 years ago at 35 weeks' gestation and spent 4 days in the hospital before discharge. She has no other risk factors for preterm labor. Vital signs (VS) are normal. Her vaginal examination was essentially within normal limits (WNL): cervix long, closed, and thick; membranes intact. Abdominal examination revealed the abdomen was nontender, with fundal height at 29 cm, fetus in a vertex presentation.

5. While you are waiting for laboratory results, what therapeutic measures do you consider?

CASE STUDY PROGRESS

Two hours later the laboratory results indicate a UTI. The contraction monitor indicates only occasional mild contractions. Her physician discharges her to home on an antibiotic for the UTI.

6. What follow-up (F/U) measures should be considered?

Case Study **117**

Name _____ Class/Group _____ Date _____
Group Members _____
INSTRUCTIONS All questions apply to this case study. Your responses should be brief and to the point. When asked to provide several answers, list them in order of priority or significance. Do not assume information that is not provided. Please print or write clearly. If your response is not legible, it will be marked as ? and you will need to rewrite it.

Scenario

J.F. is an 18-year-old single African-American woman, gravida 1 para 0, at 38 weeks' gestation. This morning in clinic she had blood pressure (BP) 142/94 mm Hg, pulse 88 beats/min, edema +2, headache, deep tendon reflexes (DTRs) +2, no clonus, proteinuria +2. Her physician is admitting her for induction of labor. She felt fine until 2 days ago, when she noticed swelling in her hands, feet, and face. She complains of a frontal headache, which started yesterday and hasn't abated with acetaminophen (Tylenol). She says she feels irritable and doesn't want the overhead lights on.

1. What other questions should you ask her at this time?

2. What information should you obtain from her obstetric record?

3. What laboratory values should be considered at this time?

4. What are three possible complications with preeclampsia?

5. Why is J.F. at risk for preeclampsia?

6. Identify eight measures that would likely be implemented.

CASE STUDY PROGRESS

J.F. progresses in labor, and at 4-cm dilation her membranes spontaneously rupture. The small amount of amniotic fluid is green, indicating the fetus has had a meconium bowel movement.

7. What does this indicate? What are the risks?

8. J.F. delivers 5 hours later a 6 pound, 8 ounce boy, with Apgar of 6 to 7. What are your responsibilities at this time?

chapter 12

Women's Health Conditions

Case Study 118

Scenario

K.W. is an 18-year-old woman who comes to Planned Parenthood for a pregnancy test because a condom broke during intercourse the night before. Her last menstrual period (LMP) was 13 days ago and was normal. She always has a monthly menstrual cycle. She is extremely nervous about pregnancy because she is beginning college on a scholarship soon. She states there have been no other acts of unprotected intercourse since her LMP. She did take oral contraceptives briefly in the past but discontinued use due to weight gain and mood swings.

1. As the RN working in the clinic, should you run a pregnancy test?

2. K.W. asks if she is at risk for pregnancy. How should you respond?

3. She asks what contraceptive options are available to her at this point. How should you answer?

4. K.W. says, "Are you talking about having an abortion?" Formulate a response.

CASE STUDY PROGRESS

There are three EC options: contraceptive pills containing estrogen and progesterone, progesterone-only pills, and the copper intrauterine device (IUD).

5. She asks you to explain the differences among the various options. What would you tell her?

6. She asks you about side effects. What would you tell her?

7. Which of the above methods of EC would you offer this patient?

8. How would you counsel this patient?

Case Study **119**

Name _____ Class/Group _____ Date _____

Group Members _____

INSTRUCTIONS All questions apply to this case study. Your responses should be brief and to the point. When asked to provide several answers, list them in order of priority or significance. Do not assume information that is not provided. Please print or write clearly. If your response is not legible, it will be marked as ? and you will need to rewrite it.

Scenario

L.W., a 20-year-old college student, comes to the clinic for a pregnancy test. She has been sexually active with her boyfriend of 6 months, and her menstrual period is now 2 weeks late. The pregnancy test is positive. The patient begins to cry saying, "I don't know what to do."

1. How would you begin to counsel L.W.?

2. What options does a woman experiencing an unplanned pregnancy have?

3. If your role is to assist her in making the choice, what information would you want L.W. to provide?

4. What are the nurse's moral and ethical obligations in this situation?

5. L.W. wants to know when she has to decide.

6. L.W. asks you if there are any actions she should be doing now to take care of herself. You would tell her:

7. L.W. asks you to tell her about abortion. What should you tell her?

8. L.W. wants you to explain the difference between vacuum aspiration and medical abortion. How would you explain this to her?

9. She tells you that she has heard that if a woman has an abortion, she may not be able to get pregnant again. How would you counsel her?

10. What type of emotional reactions do women experience after an abortion?

11. What factors affect carrying a pregnancy to term? L.W. asks you about the importance of prenatal care. Explain.

12. Finally, L.W. wants to know about adoption. What should you tell her?

Case Study **120**

Scenario

You are working in a busy OB/GYN office, and the last patient of the day is P.B., a 36-year-old who is planning to get married soon. She wants to use birth control but is not sure what to choose. Her fiancé is in law school, and they do not have health insurance, so she is anxious not to get pregnant right away. She asks you to review the various methods and help her explore what is best for her.

1. What past medical information will you need to ask P.B. about?

2. Are there any other conditions that would influence the choice of a contraceptive method?

3. Is P.B. at risk for sexually transmitted disease (STDs)?

4. What lifestyle information will help you assist P.B. in choosing an appropriate method for her?

5. P.B. asks you about the effectiveness rating of available birth control methods. Categorize your response according to the follow efficacy ratings: most effective (more than 99%), highly effective (97% to 99%), and moderately effective (less than 90%).

6. P.B. asks you to explain the main advantages and disadvantages of the most effective methods.

7. What are the main advantages and disadvantages of the contraceptive methods in the highly effective category?

8. What about the moderately effective birth control methods? What are the main advantages and disadvantages?

9. She wants to know about cost with each method because she will be on a tight budget, with limited insurance coverage.

10. She asks you which method you would pick. What do you tell her?

Case Study **121**

Scenario

You are working as the triage nurse in the emergency department (ED) at a busy tertiary care center. A woman comes in complaining of (C/O) very heavy vaginal bleeding and extreme pain. S.K. is single, is 47 years of age, and has been bleeding for 24 hours, soaking a pad an hour. She thinks her last menstrual period (LMP) was 2 months ago, but they have been irregular and she isn't sure. She has had some spotting during the past 6 months and is afraid of the amount of bleeding in the past 24 hours. She works in a law firm as a paralegal and was embarrassed yesterday when she leaked around her pad and stained a chair in the conference room. She has 2 sexual partners currently and has 2 children from a previous marriage.

1. Identify three conditions that would require emergency care and could prove life threatening.

CASE STUDY PROGRESS

You determine that S.K. is stable at the present level of bleeding; her vital signs (VS) are 110/68, 88, 22. She is not diaphoretic or pale. Her blood loss, although significant, does not have the same presentation as hemorrhage with imminent hypovolemic shock.

2. She looks horrified and asks you, "Could I be pregnant?" How should you respond?

3. S.K. reports she hasn't been using birth control because she has sex so rarely. She wants to know if a urine pregnancy test would tell her whether she is pregnant. Provide information about a urine pregnancy test.

CASE STUDY PROGRESS

You go on to explain that there are other concerns with her heavy bleeding, so an ultrasound (US) will be done to determine if she is pregnant and to exclude some of the most serious possible causes of her bleeding. You ask her how she would feel if she were pregnant, and she says, "It would ruin my life." She states she is a single mother with 2 children in junior high school.

4. What can you tell her to help her with her obvious distress?

CASE STUDY PROGRESS

You inform her that you have counselors if she needs to talk to someone. "Everything we do here today or talk about is confidential."

During her US her blood pressure (BP) drops to 90/42 mm Hg and she C/O considerable cramping. The physician asks you to start an IV and infuse 1 L of D_5LR to replace the volume lost during the last 24 hours and writes a prescription for meperidine (Demerol) 25 mg IV.

5. Before administering the meperidine, what should you ask her?

CASE STUDY PROGRESS

Her US is negative for pregnancy; she does not have an ectopic or intrauterine pregnancy. The US shows a very thick endometrial lining, even after 24 hours of bleeding.

6. S.K. is obviously relieved about not being pregnant, but while the physician is out of the cubicle writing discharge orders, she expresses fear that this could be cancer. What should you tell her to reassure her?

7. S.K. asks what she can do to keep this from happening again. Please respond.

8. What risk factors should you ask her about before discussing birth control pills as a treatment option?

9. If S.K. is prescribed birth control pills for the treatment of her bleeding problem, what other risks should she be aware of if she is using the pills for birth control?

CASE STUDY PROGRESS

S.K. is more comfortable now. The physician suggests birth control pills to control her bleeding. He tells her to take 2 pills a day for 2 or 3 days until her bleeding stops. Once the bleeding has stopped, she should continue using the medication, 1 pill/day, for the rest of the cycle.

10. What warning signs and symptoms do you want to tell her about as she starts her contraceptive pills?

CASE STUDY PROGRESS

You give her the telephone number of her OB/GYN and suggest she make the appointment right away. Reinforce that an endometrial biopsy to see if she has any abnormal cells with her heavy bleeding would be a good idea. Again, you stress she should go to her OB/GYN right away if the bleeding increases or the birth control pills do not stop her bleeding. She states that she understands.

Case Study **122**

Scenario

You are the nurse in a walk-in clinic. A.P. is being seen this morning for a 2-day history of diffuse but severe abdominal pain. She has complaints of (C/O) nausea without vomiting but denies vaginal bleeding or discharge. A.P. claims to have had unprotected sex with several partners, some of whom have penile discharge. Her last menstrual period (LMP) ended 3 days ago. She has no known drug allergies (NKDA) and denies previous medical or psychiatric problems. Vital signs (VS) are 108/60, 110, 20, 100.6° F (tympanic).

Physical examination finds her abdomen is very tender. The slightest touch of her abdomen causes her to wince with pain. Bowel sounds are normal. Pelvic examination finds purulent material pooled in the vaginal vault, which appears to be coming from the cervix. A sample of the vaginal drainage is obtained and sent for culture.

1. What medical interventions can you anticipate?

2. Based on A.P.'s stated history and the results of the vaginal examination, the physician also treats her for *Chlamydia* infection. What should you teach A.P. about her disease?

3. Based on the previous question, identify the potential issues for noncompliance and what other action might encourage successful compliance.

CASE STUDY PROGRESS

The physician has the option of treating A.P. by one of two different methods. First, the physician could prescribe treatment over a period of 1 week; A.P. would be given the first dose of doxycycline (Monodox) 100 mg PO, then would be given a prescription for the same dose to be taken PO bid for 7 days. Second, the physician could prescribe a one-time dose of azithromycin (Zithromax) 1 g PO, which could be administered in the clinic.

4. A one-time dose of azithromycin 1 g PO is ordered for A.P. Why is this a good choice for her?

5. *Chlamydia* infection is considered a sexually transmitted disease (STD) that is mandated to be reported to the public health department (PHD). Why?

6. You ask if someone has talked with A.P. about "safe sex." She laughs and tells you there is nothing safe about sex. Undaunted, you ask if she would be willing for you to discuss the use of condoms with her sexual partners. She tells you that she's already careful; if she doesn't know the guy, she uses condoms every time. How are you going to respond?

7. You ask A.P. if she has been tested for HIV. She says no, she doesn't know anyone with AIDS, and she doesn't do sex with gay men. Now what are you going to say?

8. You ask her if she would like to be tested for HIV. It won't cost her anything, and no one will know the results but her; it's completely confidential. She agrees to the test and it comes back positive. What is her prognosis?

Case Study **123**

Scenario

T.C. is a 30-year-old woman who 3 weeks ago underwent a vaginal hysterectomy and right salpingo-oophorectomy for abdominal pain and endometriosis. Postoperatively she experienced an intraabdominal hemorrhage, and her hematocrit (Hct) dropped from 40.5% to 21%. She was transfused with 3 units of packed RBCs (PRBCs). After discharge she continued to have abdominal pain, chills, and fever and was subsequently readmitted twice: once for treatment of postoperative infection and the second time for evacuation of a pelvic hematoma. Despite treatment, T.C. continued to have abdominal pain, chills, fever, and nausea and vomiting (N/V).

T.C. has now been admitted to your unit after an exploratory laparotomy. Vital signs (VS) are 130/70, 94, 16, 37.6°C (tympanic). She is easily aroused and oriented to place and person. She dozes between verbal requests. She has a low-midline abdominal dressing that is dry and intact and a Jackson-Pratt (JP) drain that is fully compressed and contains a scant amount of bright red blood. Her Foley to down drain (DD) has clear yellow urine. She has an IV of 1000 ml $D_5.45NS$ infusing at 100 ml/hr in her left forearm, with no swelling or redness. T.C. is receiving IV morphine sulfate for pain control through a patient-controlled analgesia (PCA) pump. The settings are dose 2 mg, lock-out interval 15 minutes, 4-hour maximum dose of 30 mg. When aroused, she states that her pain is an 8 on a scale of 1 to 10. She also has 2 L oxygen by nasal cannula (O_2/NC), and her Sao_2 by pulse oximeter is 93%.

1. During your assessment you note that T.C.'s respiratory rate is 16 breaths/min and shallow. Articulate your plan for a more complete assessment of T.C.s' condition. Include factors to be considered, the supporting rationale, and your actions.

CASE STUDY PROGRESS

The unit is busy when T.C. is returned from the postanesthesia care unit (PACU). Staffing is minimal. You are concerned about monitoring T.C. carefully enough. Your present patient load is 6; of these, 2 patients are newly postop and 1 is getting ready for discharge. You have a nursing assistant who helps you and another RN. You are most concerned with T.C.'s respiratory status and the possibility that she may, in her drowsy state, self-administer a dose of narcotic that would further reduce her respiratory status (despite the lock-out time).

2. Formulate a plan, given the resources mentioned previously.

3. Pain control using the PCA can be tricky. Throughout the first postop day, it has been difficult to balance T.C.'s need for pain medication and depression of her respiratory status. Discuss the concepts of controlling pain with IV narcotics and factors that may be adjusted to better control her pain.

4. T.C. is beginning to withdraw from conversations with you and the other staff. She sleeps most of the day and is not eating. At times she is tearful and is irritable with her husband. You believe that she is showing signs of depression. What actions should you take to help her?

CASE STUDY PROGRESS

T.C. and her husband are talking one evening, and you overhear that they are very dissatisfied with the care provided by the physician. They believe that he has mismanaged T.C.'s care. They are discussing getting an attorney. They ask you what you think.

5. What do you do?

6. You state, "Tell me what's going on with you right now. Maybe I can help you be more comfortable." What would be the benefit of taking this approach?

7. Mr. C. says, "No one is telling us anything. My wife came in here for a simple hysterectomy. She ends up with 4 surgeries. She still has pain, and she's worse off than when she started. Somebody has screwed up big time. Then they have the nerve to send me a bill. This morning they demanded $185,000. I'm not paying a dime until she gets better." How are you going to respond?

chapter 13

Psychiatric Disorders

Case Study 124

Scenario

You are the nurse working triage in the emergency department (ED). This afternoon a woman brings in her father, K.B., a 72-year-old. The daughter reports that over the past several months she has noticed her father has progressively had problems with his mental capacity. These changes have developed gradually but seem to be getting worse. At times he is alert, and at other times he seems disoriented, depressed, and tearful. He is forgetting things and doing things out of the ordinary, such as placing the milk in the cupboard and sugar in the refrigerator. This morning he thought it was nighttime and wondered what his daughter was doing at his house. He could not pour his own coffee, and he seems to be getting more agitated. K.B. reports that he has been having memory problems for the past year and at times has difficulty remembering the names of family members and friends.

A review of his past medical history (PMH) is significant for hypercholesterolemia and coronary artery disease (CAD). He had a myocardial infarction (MI) 5 years ago. K.B.'s vital signs (VS) today are all within normal limits (WNL).

1. What are some cognitive changes seen in a number of elderly patients?

2. You know that age-related changes in the elderly may influence cognitive functioning. Name and discuss one.

3. You understand that other disorders may have presentations similar to dementia. Identify one.

4. Identify four patient behaviors you would associate with depression.

5. What patient behaviors would you associate with delirium? Identify three.

6. What are the behaviors associated with dementia? Identify three.

7. You know that there are four main types of dementia that result in cognitive changes. List two of these types of dementia.

8. How can the level or degree of the dementia impairment be determined?

9. What neuroanatomic changes are seen in individuals with Alzheimer's disease?

10. A number of diagnostic tests have been ordered for K.B. From the tests listed below, which would be used to diagnose dementia?
- Mental status examinations
- Toxicology screen
- Mini–Mental State Examination
- ECG
- CMP
- CBC with differential
- Thyroid function tests
- Colonoscopy
- RPR
- Serum B_{12}
- Bleeding time
- HIV screening
- CT
- MRI

CASE STUDY PROGRESS
K.B. was diagnosed with Alzheimer's dementia.

11. List at least three interventions would you plan for K.B.

Available websites for additional information include:
Alzheimer's Association: *http://www.alz.org*
National Institute on Aging: *http://www.nia.nih.gov/alzheimers*

Case Study **125**

Name _____ Class/Group _____ Date _____
Group Members _____
INSTRUCTIONS All questions apply to this case study. Your responses should be brief and to the point. When asked to provide several answers, list them in order of priority or significance. Do not assume information that is not provided. Please print or write clearly. If your response is not legible, it will be marked as ? and you will need to rewrite it.

Scenario

You are working the day shift on a medicine inpatient unit. You are discussing discharge instructions with J.B., an 86-year-old man who was admitted for mitral valve repair. His serum blood glucose had been averaging 250 mg/dl or higher for the past several months. During this admission, his dosage of insulin was adjusted, and he was given additional education in managing his diet. While you are giving these instructions, J.B. tells you his wife died 9 months ago. He becomes tearful when telling you about that loss and the loneliness he has been feeling. He tells you he just doesn't feel good lately, feels sad much of the time, and hasn't been involved in his normal activities. He has few friends left in the community, since most of them have passed away. He also tells you that he has been feeling so down the past few months that he has had thoughts about suicide.

1. What other information should you ask J.B. regarding his thoughts of suicide?

2. What characteristics of J.B. put him at high risk for suicide?

3. Which psychiatric disorders can result in suicidal ideations or gestures?

4. What questions would you ask J.B. to determine whether he is clinically depressed?

5. Ill people often have trouble sleeping, experience a change in appetite, reduce their level of activity, and have thoughts of death. How can you tell the difference between old age with illness and depression?

6. List five of the most common signs of depression.

7. Identify two treatments that are available for depression.

8. J.B. was started on an SSRI such as fluoxetine (Prozac). What special instructions should you give him regarding SSRIs?

9. What advantages does ECT hold over the other treatments for depression?

10. ECT is a highly stigmatized treatment; many people are reluctant to consent to initiate treatment. What are the most common untoward effects of ECT?

11. What immediate interventions would you carry out for J.B.?

Websites for additional information include:
National Institute of Mental Health: ***http://www.nimh.nih.gov/health/topics/depression/index.shtml***
Mental Health America: ***http://www.depression-screening.org***

Case Study **126**

Scenario

You are the RN case manager in an outpatient mental health clinic. S.T. is here today for her outpatient mental health appointment. She has a diagnosis of bipolar disorder and has been stable for the past 3 years. Her last episode was one of mania that required hospitalization. She is 29 years old, married, with two children ages 2 and 4. She reports that her mood is better than it has been in a long time and she has lots of energy. When asked if she thinks this is a recurrence of mania, she says no, she just thinks that things are finally getting better.

1. What other information would be important to ask S.T.?

2. What other information would help determine whether S.T. is experiencing the onset of a manic or hypomanic episode?

3. Bipolar disorder is a disorder of mood, characterized by episodes of depression, mania, or hypomania. What symptoms might you see if S.T. is experiencing mania or hypomania? (See DSM-IV-TR: *Diagnostic and statistical manual of mental disorders,* 4th ed. [text rev], Washington, DC, 2000, American Psychiatric Association.)

4. How is hypomania different from mania?

CASE STUDY PROGRESS

Lithium is commonly used to treat bipolar disorder. S.T. has been taking lithium for several years.

5. When S.T. first started taking lithium, she would have been cautioned to report side effects. Identify five symptoms she should report.

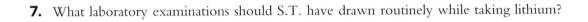

6. Lithium toxicity can occur in patients taking lithium. What are the symptoms of lithium toxicity?

7. What laboratory examinations should S.T. have drawn routinely while taking lithium?

8. What instructions should have been given to S.T when she began lithium therapy?

9. Aside from lithium, what other medications are used to treat bipolar disorder?

10. Given her history of bipolar disorder, what should you teach S.T. to minimize mood swings?

Case Study **127**

Name _____ Class/Group _____ Date _____

Group Members _____

INSTRUCTIONS All questions apply to this case study. Your responses should be brief and to the point. When asked to provide several answers, list them in order of priority or significance. Do not assume information that is not provided. Please print or write clearly. If your response is not legible, it will be marked as ? and you will need to rewrite it.

Scenario

You are working on an inpatient psychiatric unit and are to do an initial assessment on R.B., who has just been admitted. He has a diagnosis of schizophrenia, paranoid type. He is 22 years old and has been attending the local university and living at home with his parents. He has always been a good student and has been active socially. Last semester his grades began declining, and he became very withdrawn. He spends most of his time alone in his room. His grooming has deteriorated; he may go days without bathing. For several weeks before admission he insisted on keeping all of the blinds and curtains in the house closed. For the past 2 days he has refused to eat, saying, "They have contaminated the food." As you approach R.B., you note that he appears to be carrying on a conversation with someone, but there is no one there. When you talk to him, he looks around and answers in a whisper but gives you little information.

1. What are the *negative symptoms* of schizophrenia that R.B. may be experiencing? You should be able to identify at least three (DSM-IV-TR).

2. Identify one *positive symptom* of schizophrenia that R.B. is experiencing.

3. Give the definition of each of the following types of delusional thinking: thought broadcasting, thought insertion, grandiosity, ideas of reference.

4. What symptoms would indicate that R.B. has paranoid schizophrenia?

5. Why is it important to know R.B.'s history before he is diagnosed with schizophrenia?

6. What diagnostic screening would be important in evaluating R.B.?

7. What medications are commonly used to treat the symptoms of schizophrenia? Organize your answers according to typical and atypical antipsychotics.

CASE STUDY PROGRESS
R.B. is started on some typical antipsychotics. You inform R.B. and his family about the common side effects of the typical antipsychotics.

8. Identify at least four symptoms.

9. What types of psychosocial treatments may be used to treat R.B.'s schizophrenia?

10. What would be the most important initial interventions in treating R.B.?

Websites for additional information include:
National Alliance on Mental Illness: *http://www.nami.org*
Schizophrenia.com: *http://www.schizophrenia.com*

Case Study **128**

Scenario

J.M., a 23-year-old woman, was admitted to the psychiatric unit last night after assessment and treatment at a local hospital emergency department (ED) for "blacking out at school." She has been given a preliminary diagnosis of anorexia nervosa. As you begin to assess her, you notice that she has very loose clothing and is wrapped in a blanket. She tells you, "I don't know why I'm here. They're making a big deal about nothing." She appears to be extremely thin and pale, with dry and brittle hair, and she constantly complains about being cold. As you ask questions pertaining to weight and nutrition, she becomes defensive and vague, but she does admit to losing "some" weight after an appendectomy 2 years ago. She tells you that she used to be fat, but after her surgery she didn't feel like eating and everybody started commenting on how good she was beginning to look, so she just quit eating for a while. She informs you that she is eating lots now, even though everyone keeps "bugging me about my weight and how much I eat." She eventually admits to a weight loss of "about 40 pounds and I'm still fat."

1. How is the diagnosis of anorexia nervosa determined?

2. What are the clinical symptoms of anorexia nervosa? Identify eight symptoms.

3. What are concomitant disorders associated with anorexia nervosa?

4. Name behaviors that J.M. may engage in other than self-starvation.

5. What are common family dynamics with anorexia nervosa?

6. What are the clinical symptoms that should have the highest priority? Why?

7. In general, the care plans for patients with anorexia are detailed and include many psychologic aspects. What are they? You should be able to name at least 10.

CASE STUDY PROGRESS

J.M. is ready for discharge teaching, and you are assisting the RN. J.M. states, "I'll be so glad to get out of this place. I'm so fat and ugly. I need to lose 10 pounds. I bet I can do it in just a couple of days. I don't want to live anymore."

8. What will you and the RN discuss with the primary care provider (PCP) before any further discharge teaching or plans?

9. You report J.M.'s statements to the PCP. How will the treatment plan be altered?

10. What medications would be indicated for J.M. to assist with resolution of both her anorexia nervosa and major depression?

11. What would indicate successful treatment with J.M.?

Websites for additional information include:

National Alliance on Mental Illness: *http://www.nami.org/helpline/anorexia.htm*

National Association of Anorexia Nervosa and Associated Disorders: *http://www.anad.org*

National Eating Disorders Association: *http://www.edap.org*

Case Study **129**

Name _____ **Class/Group** _____ **Date** _____

Group Members _____

INSTRUCTIONS All questions apply to this case study. Your responses should be brief and to the point. When asked to provide several answers, list them in order of priority or significance. Do not assume information that is not provided. Please print or write clearly. If your response is not legible, it will be marked as ? and you will need to rewrite it.

Scenario

You are working the evening shift in an inpatient psychiatric unit. The patients are in the day room watching a movie when suddenly someone starts yelling. You and other staff rush to the day room to find J.J., a 55-year-old male patient, crouched in the corner behind a chair, yelling at the other patients, "Get down. Get down quick." You and the other staff are able to calm J.J. and the other patients and take J.J. to his room. He apologizes for his outburst and explains to you that the movie brought back memories of Vietnam. He had forgotten where he was and thought he was in combat again. He describes to you in detail the memory he had of being ambushed by the enemy and watching several of his comrades be killed. You remember hearing in report that J.J. is a Vietnam War veteran.

1. What is the most likely cause of J.J.'s behavior?

2. According to the DSM-IV-TR, name three criteria that must be present to diagnose posttraumatic stress disorder (PTSD).

3. What is the difference between PTSD and acute stress disorder, according to the DSM-IV-TR?

4. Which symptom(s) of PTSD did J.J. most likely experience?

5. What therapeutic measures could be done to help J.J. during your shift this evening?

✳ **Note:** *When a clinician is faced with a patient who has experienced a significant trauma, major treatment approaches are support; encouragement to discuss the event; and education regarding a variety of treatments, including relaxation techniques, psychotherapy, and medication.*

6. Give examples of common antianxiety agents used to sedate a person experiencing severe anxiety.

✳ **Note:** *Some anxiolytics are controlled substances and should be used with caution (e.g., benzodiazepines such as lorazepam, alprazolam, diazepam, chlordiazepoxide, and clonazepam). Note also that hydroxyzine is an effective antihistamine, and that patients over age 60 have a higher incidence of side effects and may require lower doses than younger patients.*

7. What are the adverse effects of long-term use of benzodiazepine anxiolytics?

8. What types of medications can be used safely for chronic anxiety disorders such as PTSD? Give examples of each.

9. List some relaxation techniques that could be implemented or taught to J.J. to help relieve his anxiety.

10. What other treatment modalities could J.J. be referred to after his hospitalization to help treat his PTSD and related problems?

For more information, contact the National Center for Posttraumatic Stress Disorder *(http://www. ncptsd.va.gov).*

Case Study **130**

Scenario

J.G., a 49-year-old man, was seen in the emergency department (ED) 2 days ago, diagnosed (Dx) with alcohol intoxication, and released after 8 hours to his brother's care. He was brought back to the ED 12 hours ago with an active gastrointestinal (GI) bleed and is being admitted to ICU; his diagnosis is upper GI bleed and alcohol intoxication.

You are assigned to admit and care for J.G. for the remainder of your shift. According to the ED notes, his admission vital signs (VS) were 84/56, 110, 26, and he was vomiting bright red blood. His labs were remarkable for Hct 23%, alanine transaminase (ALT) 69 IU/ml, aspartate transaminase (AST) 111 IU/ml, and serum alcohol (ETOH) 271 mg/dl. He was given IV fluids and transfused 6 units of packed RBCs (PRBCs) in the ED. On initial assessment, you note that J.G.'s VS are blood pressure (BP) 154/90 mm Hg, pulse 98 beats/min; he has a slight tremor in his hands, and he appears anxious. He complains of a headache and appears flushed. You note that he has not had any emesis and has not had any frank red blood in his stool or "black tarry stools" over the past 5 hours. In response to your questions, J.G. denies that he has an alcohol problem but later admits to drinking approximately a fifth of vodka daily for the past 2 months. He reports having been drinking just before his admission to the ED. He admits to having had seizures while withdrawing from alcohol in the past.

1. Which data from your assessment of J.G. are of concern to you?

2. What are two most likely causes of J.G.'s symptoms?

3. What is the most likely time frame for someone to have withdrawal symptoms after abrupt cessation of alcohol?

CASE STUDY PROGRESS
You note that J.G.'s physician has not diagnosed J.G. as having alcohol dependence, and his orders do not include treatment for alcohol withdrawal.

4. As an RN, what action is necessary before you continue to care for J.G.?

5. According to the DSM-IV-TR, what is the difference between alcohol dependence and alcohol abuse?

6. What would be helpful for J.G.'s physician to know regarding J.G.'s substance abuse history?

7. Which clinical assessment tool is commonly used to monitor withdrawal symptoms? Explain how it is used.

8. What medications are commonly prescribed for patients withdrawing from alcohol?

9. What chronic health problems are associated with alcoholism?

10. What other medical problems will J.G.'s physician need to be aware of as he provides J.G.'s treatment for alcohol withdrawal? How could you help assess for these problems?

11. What lab tests might the physician order to assess for nutritional deficiencies or other medical problems J.G. is experiencing?

12. What types of education and referral should be done before J.G.'s discharge from the hospital?

13. What medications might be prescribed to J.G. to assist him with sobriety? What is the usual treatment regimen, and what side effects and precautions should you educate the patient about concerning each?

Websites for additional information include:

National Institute on Alcohol Abuse and Alcoholism: *http://www.niaaa.nih.gov*

National Clearinghouse for Alcohol and Drug Information: *http://ncadi.samhsa.gov*

Case Study **131**

Scenario

It is 1000 hours in the emergency department (ED) when the ambulance brings in G.G., a 35-year-old
man who is having difficulty breathing. He complains of (C/O) chest pain and tightness, dizziness, palpitations, nausea, paresthesia, and feelings of impending doom and unreality; he is having trouble
thinking clearly. He tells you, "I don't think I'm going to make it. I must be having a heart attack." He
is diaphoretic and trembling. His vital signs (VS) are 184/92, 104, 28, 98.4° F. This episode began at
work during a meeting at approximately 0920 and became progressively worse. A co-worker called
911 and stayed with the patient until medical help arrived. The patient has no history of cardiac
problems.

1. What would the highest medical priorities be for G.G.?

CASE STUDY PROGRESS

After a full medical work-up, it is determined that G.G. is stable. His shortness of breath (SOB) and
anxiety are resolved after giving lorazepam 1 mg IV push (IVP). There is no evidence of any physical
disorder, and the diagnosis of panic attack has been made. G.G. admits to having had 3 similar episodes
in the past 2 weeks; however, they were not nearly as severe or long lasting.

2. How do you think this diagnosis was determined?

3. G.G. asks if there is something wrong with his memory because he has been having
trouble remembering things. What effect does panic disorder have on memory?

CASE STUDY PROGRESS

G.G. shares with the ED staff that he has been under severe stress at work and home. He tells them he is going through a divorce, he lost a child last summer in a motor vehicle accident (MVA), and his company is downsizing. He will probably be out of a job soon. He hasn't been sleeping well for the past couple of months and has lost about 20 pounds.

4. Identify five additional triggers that could cause anxiety to build to the point of panic.

5. G.G. wants to know what causes panic attacks or disorder. Using etiologic theories regarding anxiety, what will you tell him?

6. G.G. has questions regarding the differences between panic attacks and panic disorder. According to the DSM-IV-TR, what are the differences?

7. What medications are used to treat panic attacks? What will your patient teaching include?

8. G.G. expresses fear of panic attacks returning and wants to know what techniques would help him cope.

9. What is systematic desensitization?

10. What actions or interventions are most indicated in the treatment of panic disorder?

11. G.G. wants to know how he will be able to tell if he is successfully managing his anxiety disorder. What should you tell him?

Websites for additional information include:
Medline Plus: *http://medlineplus.gov*
National Panic & Anxiety Disorder News: *http://www.npadnews.com*

chapter 14

Alternative Therapies

Case Study **132**

Name		Class/Group	Date

Group Members _____

INSTRUCTIONS All questions apply to this case study. Your responses should be brief and to the point. When asked to provide several answers, list them in order of priority or significance. Do not assume information that is not provided. Please print or write clearly. If your response is not legible, it will be marked as ? and you will need to rewrite it.

Scenario

J.B., a 45-year-old woman, is an office manager for a busy law firm and single mother of 2 children. While cleaning a shower stall, she experienced a sharp pain in her lower back. Over the next few hours her lower back became increasingly more painful. By the time she picked up the children from their sporting event and drove to the nearest walk-in medical clinic, she had a sharp shooting pain into her right buttocks. Her spinal x-rays were not significant, and she was diagnosed with acute musculoskeletal strain and given antiinflammatories, hydrocodone 5 mg/acetaminophen 500 mg (Lortab) PO q6h prn for pain, and instructed to rest her back for the next 24 hours. Monday morning she called in sick to work because she couldn't think clearly because of the pain medication. She developed stomach pain, and her back pain was only slightly improved. She called a friend who had experienced a similar episode and related a favorable outcome after being treated with acupuncture. J.B. comes to your alternative medicine clinic for her acupuncture appointment.

1. As you complete her intake interview, she asks, "What is acupuncture?" What would you tell her?

2. J.B. wants to know how acupuncture works. How should you explain acupuncture to her?

3. J.B. asks how acupuncture can help her back pain. Explain how acupuncture differs from traditional Western medicine in the treatment of back pain.

4. J.B. asks, "What does it feel like? Does it hurt?" How should you respond?

5. J.B. asks, "Does insurance cover the cost?" Provide a response.

6. List possible risks and complications of acupuncture.

7. What types of condition can be treated with acupuncture?

8. J.B. asks where she could find an acupuncture practitioner.

Case Study **133**

Scenario

One month ago J.P., a 50-year-old man, came to the outpatient clinic with complaints of (C/O) mild shortness of breath (SOB) and some mild intermittent chest pain. He described himself as a high-stress, type A personality who owns his own business and works long hours. He has smoked 1 pack of cigarettes per day (PPD) for the past 30 years. He has tried to quit several times and was successful for as long as 6 months at a time, but when business became stressful, he started smoking again. Also, J.P. said he has been trying to lose the extra 30 pounds he is carrying but stated it is difficult to exercise due to the long hours of work. The cardiac work-up is negative for coronary artery disease (CAD), and he has returned for a follow-up (F/U) visit. During the discussion about lifestyle changes, J.P. expresses interest in medical hypnosis for stress management, smoking cessation, and weight loss. He would like more information. You are the case manager for the clinic and meet with J.P. to discuss medical hypnosis.

1. J.P. asks, "What is hypnosis?" What should you tell him?

2. J.P. asks what you mean by *trance state*. Explain the term.

3. J.P. wants to know what you mean by *subconscious mind*. Explain.

4. J.P. asks, "How does hypnosis work to help someone change a subconscious belief?"

5. J.P. states he has seen TV shows where people did silly things on stage. He wants to know how medical hypnosis is different from TV hypnosis. Explain.

6. J.P. asks how you can tell if hypnosis will work for a patient. Please respond.

7. J.P. wants to know how hypnosis is done and what happens during a session. You inform him that medical hypnosis has several components: patient preparation and education, establishing a rapport and trusting relationship, induction and deepening, hypnotic suggestions, and reawakening from the trance state. Briefly explain each step.

8. J.P asks what types of medical conditions can be helped by hypnosis. How should you respond?

9. J.P. asks if hypnosis is contraindicated for anyone. Please respond.

10. J.P. apologizes for being full of questions but wants to know if hypnosis can be done in a group or if it is one on one. Please respond.

11. J.P asks how he would go about finding a hypnotist. Formulate an answer.

For more information contact:

American Psychological Association: Division 30, Society of Psychological Hypnosis, 750 First Street NE, Washington, DC 20002-4242; *http://www.apa.org/divisions/div30*

American Society of Clinical Hypnosis: 140 N. Bloomingdale Road, Bloomingdale, IL 60108; (630) 980-4740; info@asch.net; *http://www.asch.net*

National Board for Certified Clinical Hypnotherapists: 1110 Fidler Lane, Suite 1218, Silver Springs, MD 20901; (800) 449-8144; admin@natboard.com; *http://www.natboard.com*

Recommended journals include:

American Journal of Clinical Hypnosis: C/O American Society of Clinical Hypnosis, 140 N. Bloomingdale Road, Bloomingdale, IL 60108; (630) 980-4740; *http://asch.net/ajch.htm*

International Journal of Clinical and Experimental Hypnosis: Sage Publications, 2455 Teller Road, Thousand Oaks, CA 91320; (805) 499-9774; *http://www.ijceh.com*

Multiple System Disorders

Case Study **134**

Scenario

You are working the day shift on the medical-surgical unit in a small rural community hospital. Your assignment includes an 18-year-old woman, A.N., admitted the previous night. A.N. was caught in a house fire and sustained burns over 30% of her body surface area, with partial-thickness burns on her legs and back.

1. A.N. is undergoing burn fluid resuscitation using the standard Baxter (Parkland) formula. She was burned at 0200 and admitted at 0400. She weighs 110 pounds. Calculate her fluid requirements, specify the fluids used in the Baxter (Parkland) formula, specify how much will be given, and indicate what time intervals will be used.

   ✳ **Note:** *Addition of vitamin C to IV fluids is not part of the standard Baxter (Parkland) formula. However, depending on the preferences of the treating physician, at the onset of treatment, IV fluids containing 25 mg/ml vitamin C may be ordered to promote healing. Following is a brief summary of the pros and cons of using antioxidants in burn patient fluid resuscitation.*

   A great deal of interest exists in using antioxidants as adjuncts to resuscitation to try to minimize oxidant-mediated contributions to the inflammatory cascade. In particular, megadose vitamin C infusion during resuscitation has been studied at some length. Some animal models have demonstrated that infusion of vitamin C within 6 hours postburn can lower calculated resuscitation values by up to one half. Whether this phenomenon can be reproduced successfully in human subjects has not been clearly demonstrated.

   Proponents have reached no consensus regarding the proper total dose. Some have adopted the strategy of placing up to 10 g in a liter of RL solution, infusing it at 100 ml/hr (1 g/hr vitamin C), and counting the volume as part of the resuscitation volume. Recently published data using an infusion of 66 mg/kg/hr during the first 24 hours demonstrate a 45% decrease in the required fluid resuscitation in a small group of patients.

The safety of high-dose vitamin C has been established in humans, at least for the short-term, but this strategy is probably less safe in patients who are pregnant, those with renal failure, and those with a history of oxalate kidney stones (http://www.emedicine.com/plastic/topic159.htm).

2. A.N. was sleeping when the fire started and managed to make her way out of the house through thick smoke. You are concerned about possible smoke inhalation. What assessment findings would corroborate this concern?

3. A.N. is concerned about visible scars. What will you tell her to allay her fears?

4. A.N. is in severe pain. What is the drug of choice for pain relief following burn injury, and how should it be given?

5. A.N.'s burns are to be treated by the open method with topical application of silver sulfadiazine (Silvadene). What is the major drawback to this method of treatment?

6. A special burn diet is ordered for A.N. She has always gained weight easily and is concerned about the size of the portions. What diet-related teaching will you provide?

7. Tissues under and around A.N.'s burns are severely swollen. She looks at you with tears in her eyes and asks, "Will they stay this way?" What is your answer?

8. After significant burn injury, the patient is at high risk for infection. What measures will you institute to prevent this?

9. A.N. has one area of circumferential burns on her right lower leg. What complication is she in danger of developing, and how will you monitor for it?

9. You would like to teach J.L. some practical things she can do to protect herself from infection. List five.

✱ **Hint:** *This list should include many of the same things cancer patients on chemotherapy are taught.*

Case Study **136**

Scenario

You are working evenings on an orthopedic floor. One of your patients, J.O., is a 25-year-old man who was a new admission on day shift. He was involved in a motor vehicle accident (MVA) during a high-speed police chase. His admitting diagnosis is status post (S/P) open reduction and internal fixation (ORIF) of the right femur (which was performed with the patient under general anesthesia), multiple rib fractures, sternal bruises, and multiple abrasions. He speaks some English but is more comfortable with his native language. He is under arrest for narcotics trafficking, so one wrist is shackled to the bed and a guard is stationed outside his room continuously. Another drug dealer has told him he's "coming to get him." Hospital security is aware of the situation.

Your initial assessment reveals stable vital signs (VS) of 116/78, 84, 16, 98.6° F. His only complaint is pain, for which he has a patient-controlled analgesia (PCA) pump. You note crackles in the lung bases bilaterally. His abdomen is soft and nontender. He has a nasogastric tube (NGT) connected to continuous low wall suction (LWS). His IV of D_5LR is infusing in the proximal port of a left subclavian triple-lumen catheter; the remaining 2 ports are heparin-locked. His right femur is connected to skeletal traction. The dressing is dry and intact over the incision site.

1. J.O. has not had a cigarette since the accident. He is irate because the day nurse would not let him smoke. What is your major concern about J.O.'s smoking?

2. Do you think J.O. would be a good candidate for a nicotine patch? Why or why not? State your rationale.

3. J.O.'s right leg is connected to 10 pounds of skeletal traction. As you troubleshoot the system, you note that the ropes are intact and in the tracks of the pulleys, the right leg is slightly flexed at the knee, the leg is 6 inches above the mattress, and the 10-pound weight is resting on the floor. Are any of these findings of concern to you? If so, how would you fix it?

CASE STUDY PROGRESS

The nurse in the emergency department (ED) phones to tell you that J.O.'s immunization status could not be determined when he arrived, so no tetanus immunization was given. When you ask J.O. the date of his last tetanus shot, you find out that he was born and raised in Colombia and immigrated to the United States 5 years ago. He does not know if he has ever had a tetanus shot. You inform the physician, and he orders diphtheria/tetanus toxoid 0.5 ml IM and tetanus immune globulin (HyperTET) 250 units deep IM.

4. Why is J.O. getting two injections?

5. J.O. has a Foley catheter inserted to drain his urine. What should the nurse assess for in relation to the Foley catheter?

6. While assessing distal to the fractured femur, the nurse notes that his toes are cold to the touch. What other assessment findings should be gathered?

7. J.O. has an antiembolism stocking ordered for his left leg. What is the rationale for putting stockings on only one leg?

CASE STUDY PROGRESS

At 1800 J.O.'s guard summons you to his room. J.O. is cold and clammy, pale, slightly confused, and moaning. VS are 70/palp, 140, 28, 98.0°F. His pulse is weak and thready. His abdomen is painful and appears to be distended.

8. You summon the physician. What else can you do?

9. The physician arrives and wishes to perform a peritoneal lavage. Explain why peritoneal lavage is being done, and describe the procedure.

10. What are the nurse's responsibilities in preparation for this procedure (in order)?

11. The physician begins the diagnostic peritoneal lavage procedure. On insertion of the trocar into the abdomen, bright red blood under pressure returns. What happens next?

12. In view of the threat made on J.O.'s life and his vulnerable situation, what precautions should the nursing unit take to protect him?

CASE STUDY PROGRESS

J.O. recovered for several weeks in the hospital before being sent to jail to await trial. Shortly before his trial date, he was found stabbed to death in his cell. Although there was an investigation, the murder weapon was never found, and no one was ever charged in his death.

Case Study **137**

Scenario

You are working on a telemetry unit and have just received a transfer from the ICU. The 50-year-old male patient, T.A., had a repair of an abdominal aortic aneurysm (AAA) measuring 8 cm in diameter. This is his second postoperative day. He is an attorney with an active practice. Although he routinely took medication for gastritis before surgery, T.A. considered himself to be healthy before diagnosis of the aneurysm. In addition to these problems, T.A. has a 10-year history of type 2 diabetes mellitus (DM), and he has required insulin the past 6 months to control his glucose levels; he has also experienced progressive weakness of his lower extremities and decreasing urinary output since surgery.

1. T.A. has questions about his surgery. He asks you, "I was fine before surgery. I'd still be fine now if I hadn't been operated on, wouldn't I?" Based on your knowledge of AAA, what should your response be?

   ✷ **Note:** *Repair of an AAA requires the application of an aortic clamp above and below the aneurysm during the most crucial part of the surgery. Nerve damage to the legs and the formation of blood clots are risks with this surgery and require frequent assessment.*

2. You are performing your initial assessment of T.A.'s legs. What findings should you record?

3. Four hours after admission to your floor, you note that T.A. has had a urinary output of 75 ml of dark amber urine. You examine the catheter and tubing for obstructions, and there are none. What other assessment data should you gather to determine whether a problem exists?

4. Laboratory tests reveal renal damage. T.A. is placed on fluid restriction and a renal diet. T.A. asks what he is going to be able to eat on his diet. What is your reply?

5. T.A. has a dialysis catheter inserted into his left subclavian vein. You are preparing to administer an IV antibiotic and find that his only other IV access, a peripheral line, is obstructed. What should you do?

CASE STUDY PROGRESS

On return from his first dialysis, T.A. complains of (C/O) headache and nausea. He is restless and slightly confused, and he has an elevated blood pressure (BP). You suspect disequilibrium phenomenon. You notify the physician.

6. What measures can you institute at this point?

✱ **7.** T.A. has an episode of severe vomiting. His abdominal wound dehisces, and a loop of his intestines eviscerates. Another staff member has summoned the physician. What care should you render before the physician's arrival?

CASE STUDY PROGRESS

T.A. returns from the OR. You note that his blood glucose levels have ranged from 62 to 387 mg/dl over the last 7 days.

8. A sliding scale with regular insulin has been ordered. He comments, "That's funny, you're giving me about the same amount of insulin that I give myself at home. I don't understand why it's not working." How should you respond?

9. T.A.'s wound is not healing. Explain the relationship between his blood glucose readings and wound healing.

Case Study **138**

Scenario

You are a nurse working in the medical ICU and take the following report from the emergency department (ED) RN: "We have a patient for you; R.L. is an 82-year-old frail woman who has been in a nursing
home. Her admitting diagnosis [Dx] is sepsis, pneumonia, and dehydration, and she has a stage III
pressure ulcer. Past medical history [PMH] includes remote cerebrovascular accident [CVA] with residual
right-sided weakness and paresthesia, remote myocardial infarction [MI], and peripheral vascular
disease [PVD]. Her vital signs [VS] are 98/62, 88 and regular, 38 and labored, 100.4° F. Labs have been
drawn and are pending; she has oxygen [O$_2$] at 10 L via face mask, an IV of D$_5$.45NS at 100 ml/hr, and
an indwelling Foley. The infectious disease doctors have been notified, and respiratory therapy is with
the patient—they are just leaving the ED and should arrive shortly."

1. Knowing that R.L. is frail and has right–sided weakness and pressure ulcer, what consults
   would you initiate?

2. As you conduct your skin assessment, what areas of the patient's body will you pay
   particular attention to?

CASE STUDY PROGRESS

During your admission skin assessment you note that she has very dry, thin, almost transparent skin.
There are several areas of ecchymosis on her upper extremities.

3. What interventions would you initiate to prevent further skin breakdown?

4. What does it mean to "stage a pressure ulcer"?

5. What factors increase risk for the development of tissue breakdown and the formation of pressure-induced ulcers?

✳ **Note:** *Many facilities have a policy for using a validated risk assessment tool, such as Braden, Norton, or Gosnell scale, when a patient is admitted to their facility. All facilities have protocols dictating frequency of skin assessment.*

6. What are the advantages of using a validated risk assessment tool to document the patient's skin condition on admission?

7. What does a stage I pressure ulcer look like?

8. What tissues are involved in stage II through IV ulcers?

9. What are the limitations or restrictions of staging pressure ulcers?

CASE STUDY PROGRESS

As you proceed with the assessment, an enterostomal therapy (ET) and wound nurse specialist comes in. She knows R.L. from a prior admission and had ordered a specialty mattress as soon as she received the wound-bed consult. She states she has ordered an air overlay and it should be delivered to your unit before your shift ends.

10. Why is a specialty bed or mattress used for immobile or compromised patients?

✶ **Note:** *There are classifications of specialty beds and mattresses, with general guidelines for placement based on a patient's condition and risks. At one end of the spectrum are foam mattresses and gel overlays. Then there are several types of air overlays and beds: static air, dynamic air, low air loss, and fluidized air. Often they are referred to in terms of pressure relief or reduction.*

11. What are the essential points all nurses should know about the patient's bed?

12. Why do patients placed on a specialty mattresses or beds remain at risk for breakdown?

13. Why do the heels have the greatest incidence of breakdown, even when the patient is on the most advanced specialty bed?

14. What intervention can you initiate to protect R.L.'s heels?

15. R.L. has limited mobility secondary to her stroke. Her current illness may have further compromised her mobility and activity. What measures should you include in her care plan?

16. What risk factor does the drawsheet prevent or minimize?

✳ **Note:** *Pressure, friction, and shear are all mechanical injuries. Shear is a force applied parallel to the plane of an object but in the opposite direction to the force being applied. Shear is the result of gravity and resistance. For example, the head of the bed (HOB) is elevated, and the patient slowly slides toward the foot of the bed. The skin of the sacrum meets the resistance of the bed surface while gravity pulls the patient's body toward the foot of the bed. This means the skin and the bones are going in opposite directions, thereby pulling and stretching tissue and distorting vessels within the area, causing destruction of both. Undermining is thought to be the direct result of shear insult to pressure-induced injury. Friction can happen without shear, but shear always begins with friction.*

17. What intervention is needed to reduce the possibility of shear?

CASE STUDY PROGRESS

The wound nurse gently removes the old dressing, using the push-pull method and adhesive remover wipes. After she takes off the outside dressing, often called a *secondary dressing,* she pulls out the primary dressing and tells you it was "packed" too hard.

18. What problems can packing a wound too full create?

CASE STUDY PROGRESS

You maintain R.L.'s position while the wound nurse assesses the sacral pressure ulcer. The nurse confirms that the patient has a stage III pressure ulcer. As the wound nurse follows protocol to culture the wound, she is careful to avoid any cross-contamination of tissue.

19. What is considered the best-practice protocol for swab culture?

CASE STUDY PROGRESS

After she cultures the wound, you watch the nurse do a systematic assessment of the wound as per the recommended guidelines provided by the AHRQ and NPUAP. The wound nurse will chart the findings and make recommendations for management.

chapter 16

Emergency Situations

Case Study **139**

Name _____ Class/Group _____ Date _____
Group Members _____
INSTRUCTIONS All questions apply to this case study. Your responses should be brief and to the point. When asked
to provide several answers, list them in order of priority or significance. Do not assume information that is not provided.
Please print or write clearly. If your response is not legible, it will be marked as ? and you will need to rewrite it.

Scenario

You are on duty in the emergency department (ED) when a "code blue" is called overhead. As the
code nurse, you grab the crash cart and run to the code, which is in the employee lounge of the
operating room (OR). On the couch you find a nurse, Z.H., unconscious, cyanotic, and barely breathing.
Her scrub shirt has been cut off, and you attach ECG leads to her chest. Her pulse is 45 beats/min;
respirations are 8 breaths/min and shallow. She is intubated; an IV line is started with 0.9% normal
saline (NS); and she is given an ampule of 50 ml D_5W, 0.4 mg naloxone (Narcan), and 0.5 mg atropine
IV push (IVP). Her respirations improve slightly, and pulse increases to 56 beats/min. She is transported
to the ED.

1. What is the purpose of giving the three drugs mentioned in this case?

CASE STUDY PROGRESS

After additional naloxone, the patient wakes up and is extubated.

2. What additional information do you want to know?

3. In response to your questions, Z.H. tells you that she took fentanyl (Duragesic) IM. She then asks you to call a friend to come stay with her. What information would you give her friend over the phone?

4. The friend asks you what is wrong. How do you respond?

5. Identify four problems relating to Z.H.'s care that apply to this situation.

CASE STUDY PROGRESS

Z.H. is admitted to the ICU for 24-hour observation and then transferred to the chemical dependency unit.

6. What is chemical dependency?

CASE STUDY PROGRESS

One of Z.H.'s colleagues calls on the phone to ask how she is. She tells you that she thought something was wrong with Z.H. because her behavior was so erratic, but "I had no idea it was drugs. I didn't think Z.H. would ever do anything like that!" Keep in mind that patient confidentiality extends to health care professionals not directly involved in Z.H.'s care. You cannot give information on how Z.H. is doing. (For more information see Health Insurance Portability and Accountability Act [HIPAA] guidelines.)

7. What is the profile of an impaired nurse? List five characteristics.

8. What four problems are associated with impaired nurses who are practicing?

9. Z.H. asks her nurse what is going to happen to her career. What are the regulatory issues related to (R/T) impaired nurses that will guide your response? (List at least five.)

CASE STUDY PROGRESS

Z.H. successfully completes treatment and continues to practice as a nurse. She is now serving as a sponsor for another nurse undergoing treatment for chemical dependency.

Case Study **140**

Scenario

You are the nurse on a medical unit taking care of a 40-year-old man, A.A., who has been admitted with peptic ulcer disease (PUD) secondary to chronic alcoholism. He also has a history of "street" drug abuse. You enter A.A.'s room and find him having a generalized convulsive (tonic-clonic) seizure.

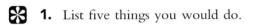 **1.** List five things you would do.

✷ **Note:** *Placing any objects, including an airway, into the patient's mouth, at this point, is contraindicated because of the possibility of patient or caregiver harm.*

CASE STUDY PROGRESS

A.A.'s seizure activity does not appear to be subsiding, and he is becoming cyanotic. The physician is notified and orders lorazepam (Ativan) 4 mg IV over 2 to 5 minutes, repeat once in 10 to 15 minutes prn.

2. What is the rationale for giving A.A. lorazepam?

3. What is status epilepticus?

4. List one thing you would be particularly alert for when giving lorazepam intravenously.

CASE STUDY PROGRESS

By the time the physician arrives, A.A.'s seizure activity has not subsided. The physician administers an additional 4 mg of lorazepam, without effect. Fifteen minutes have elapsed since you found A.A. having seizure activity.

5. What is the significance of this time lapse?

6. The physician decides to administer succinylcholine (Anectine) and intubate A.A. to protect his airway. What is succinylcholine, and why is it being administered to A.A.?

7. A.A. has been intubated; the physician orders a phenytoin (Dilantin) 20 mg/kg IV loading dose to be given at a rate of 50 mg/min, and he is transported to the ICU. What is the rationale behind giving phenytoin?

8. List two potential problems related to A.A.'s condition that could occur secondary to his current seizure activity.

9. Given A.A.'s history, state at least two possible causes for his tonic-clonic seizure.

CASE STUDY PROGRESS
A.A.'s seizure is successfully treated with lorazepam and phenytoin, and he has no further seizure activity. As you are writing up his discharge papers, you overhear A.A. telling his girlfriend to have his car brought to the hospital so he can drive home.

10. How should you respond to this situation?

Case Study **141**

Name _____ Class/Group_____ Date _____

Group Members _____

INSTRUCTIONS All questions apply to this case study. Your responses should be brief and to the point. When asked to provide several answers, list them in order of priority or significance. Do not assume information that is not provided. Please print or write clearly. If your response is not legible, it will be marked as ? and you will need to rewrite it.

Scenario

You are working on the intermediate cardiac care unit in a large hospital. You are taking care of R.J., who was admitted for a chest contusion he sustained in an auto accident; he fractured the fourth and fifth ribs on his left side. At about 2000 hours, his wife runs up to you at the nurses' station and says, "I think my husband just had a heart attack. Come quick!" She follows you into his room, where you find him face down on the floor. He is breathing and is cyanotic from the neck up. His pulse is very weak.

1. What should your first action be?

2. Suddenly, you remember R.J.'s wife, who is anxiously hovering over you in the room. What are you going to do?

CASE STUDY PROGRESS

The code team arrives. R.J.'s trauma surgeon is making rounds on your unit when the code is called, and he runs to the room. R.J. is intubated, and the normal saline (NS) lock is changed to an IV of lactated Ringer's (LR). The trauma surgeon recognizes Beck's triad and calls for a cardiac needle and syringe. He inserts the needle below the xiphoid process and aspirates 50 ml of unclotted blood.

3. What is Beck's triad, and what causes it?

4. Explain the rationale for the surgeon performing a pericardiocentesis.

CASE STUDY PROGRESS

R.J. is transferred to the thoracic ICU (TICU) for observation.

5. As the team prepares R.J.'s transfer, you go to find R.J.'s wife to thank her for alerting you to the emergency so promptly and to tell her what has happened. Briefly, and in lay terms, how would you explain what happened to her husband?

6. As you both get up to leave, Mrs. J. suddenly turns pale and says she feels very dizzy. What are you going to do?

Case Study **142**

Name _____ Class/Group _____ Date _____
Group Members _____
INSTRUCTIONS All questions apply to this case study. Your responses should be brief and to the point. When asked
to provide several answers, list them in order of priority or significance. Do not assume information that is not provided.
Please print or write clearly. If your response is not legible, it will be marked as ? and you will need to rewrite it.

Scenario

You are the nurse on duty on the intermediate care unit, and you are scheduled to take the next admission. The emergency department (ED) nurse calls to give you the following report: "This is Barb in the ED, and we have a 42-year-old man, K.L., with lower GI [gastrointestinal] bleeding. He is a sandblaster with a 12-year history of silicosis. He is taking 40 mg of prednisone per day. During the night he developed severe diarrhea. He was unable to get out of bed fast enough and had a large maroon-colored stool [hematochezia] in the bed. His wife 'freaked' and called the paramedics. He is coming to you. His vital signs [VS] are stable—110/64, 110, 28—and he's a little agitated. His temperature is 36.8°C. He hasn't had any stools since admission, but his rectal exam was guaiac positive and he is pale but not diaphoretic. We have him on 5 L O$_2$/NC [oxygen by nasal cannula]. We started a 16-gauge IV with lactated Ringer's [LR] at 125 ml/hr. He has an 18-gauge Salem sump to continuous low suction; the drainage is guaiac positive. We have done a CBC with differential, chem 14, PT/INR and PTT, a T&C [type and crossmatch] for 4 units RBCs, and a urinalysis [UA]. He's all ready for you."

1. How should you prepare for this patient's arrival?

CASE STUDY PROGRESS

K.L. arrives on your unit. As you help him transfer from the ED stretcher to the bed, K.L. becomes very dyspneic and expels 800 ml of maroon stool.

2. What are the first three actions you should take?

CASE STUDY PROGRESS

K.L. reports that he is getting nauseated but not thirsty. VS are 106/68, 116, 32.

3. What additional interventions would you need to institute?

CASE STUDY PROGRESS

Arterial blood gas (ABG) results are as follows (these results reflect values at sea level): pH 7.45, $Paco_2$ 33 mm Hg, Pao_2 65 mm Hg, HCO_3 23 mmol/L, base excess [BE] +1.0, Sao_2 91%.

4. Interpret the preceding ABGs. What do they tell you?

CASE STUDY PROGRESS

The gastroenterologist is notified by K.L.'s physician and arrives on the unit to perform a colonoscopy and endoscopy. You are going to give K.L. midazolam (Versed) and morphine sulfate IV during the procedures.

5. Given the above history, what do you think significantly contributed to the GI bleed?

6. What are midazolam and morphine sulfate, and why are they being given to K.L.?

CASE STUDY PROGRESS

During the colonoscopy, K.L. begins passing large amounts of bright red blood. He becomes more pale and diaphoretic and begins to have an altered level of consciousness (LOC).

7. Identify five immediate interventions you should initiate.

CASE STUDY PROGRESS

K.L. has been stabilized with fluids, blood, and fresh frozen plasma (FFP). There has been no further evidence of active bleeding. He received esomeprazole (Nexium) 40 mg IV push (IVP) and is placed on 40 mg PO bid.

8. Later, when he seems to be feeling better, K.L. tells you he's really embarrassed about the mess he made for you. How are you going to respond to him?

CASE STUDY PROGRESS

The physician concludes that the GI hemorrhage was prednisone induced. The prednisone is being used to suppress the progression of silicosis. The physician will discharge K.L. and attempt to decrease his maintenance dose of prednisone while monitoring his respiratory status.

Case Study **143**

Scenario

J.R. is a 28-year-old man who was doing home repairs. He fell from the top of a 6-foot stepladder, striking his head on a large rock. He experienced momentary loss of consciousness. By the time his neighbor got to him, he was conscious but bleeding profusely from a laceration over the right temporal area. The neighbor drove him to the emergency department (ED) of your hospital. As the nurse, you immediately apply a cervical collar, lay him on a stretcher, and take J.R. to a treatment room.

1. Describe the term *primary head injury*.

2. Describe a secondary head injury.

3. What steps should you take to assess J.R.?

4. List at least five components of a neurologic examination.

5. What is the most sensitive indicator of neurologic change?

CASE STUDY PROGRESS

You complete your neurologic examination and find the following: Glasgow Coma Scale (GCS) 15; pupils equal, round, react to light (PERRL); and full sensation intact. J.R. complains of (C/O) a headache and is becoming increasingly drowsy. As the radiology technician performs a portable cross-table lateral cervical spine (C-spine) x-ray, J.R. begins to speak incoherently and appears to drift off to sleep.

6. What is the next action you would take?

CASE STUDY PROGRESS

You find J.R. has become unresponsive to verbal stimuli and responds to painful stimuli by abnormally flexing his extremities (decorticate movement). He has no verbal response. The right pupil is larger than the left and does not respond to light.

7. What is J.R.'s GCS score at this time? Indicate what this means.

8. Based on his GCS score, what are the next steps you should take? The physician already has been summoned.

9. What is a normal ICP, and why is increased ICP so clinically important?

10. Identify at least five signs and symptoms (S/S) of increased ICP.

11. The physician orders a 25% mannitol solution IV. What is mannitol, and why is it being used on J.R.?

CASE STUDY PROGRESS

J.R. is transported to radiology for a CT, where he is found to have a large epidural hematoma on the right with a hemispheric shift to the left. He will be taken straight to the operating room (OR) for evacuation of the hematoma. While en route from the CT scan to the OR, the physician instructs the respiratory therapist to initiate hyperventilation of the patient to "blow off more CO_2."

12. What is the rationale for this action?

13. While he is in surgery, J.R.'s family arrives at the ED with their faith healer. They ask that their faith healer anoint J.R. and pray over him. What should the nurse say?

14. After J.R.'s surgery he is admitted to the ICU. List four medication classifications that the ICU nurse could use to decrease or control increased ICP.

15. Explain at least eight interventions you would use to prevent increased ICP in the first 48 postoperative hours.

Case Study **144**

Scenario

You are working in an outpatient clinic when a mother brings in her 20-year-old daughter, C.J., who has type 1 diabetes mellitus (DM) and has just returned from a trip to Mexico. She's had a 3-day fever and diarrhea with nausea and vomiting (N/V). She has been unable to eat and has tolerated only sips of fluid. Because she has been unable to eat, she has not taken her insulin.

Because C.J. is unsteady, you bring her to the examining room in a wheelchair. While assisting her onto the examining table, you note that her skin is warm and flushed. Her respirations are deep and rapid, and her breath is fruity smelling. C.J. is drowsy and unable to answer your questions. Her mother states, "She keeps telling me she's so thirsty, but she can't keep anything down."

1. List four pieces of additional information you need to elicit from C.J.'s mother.

CASE STUDY PROGRESS

The mother tells you the following:

"Blood glucose monitor has been reading 'high'" (some glucometers do not read above 400 mg/dl).

"C.J. has had sips of ginger ale but that's all."

"She has been vomiting about every other time she drinks."

"When she first got home, she went [voided] a lot, but yesterday she hardly went at all, and I don't think she has gone today."

"She went to bed early last night, and I could hardly wake her up this morning. That's why I brought her in."

2. Describe the pathophysiology of diabetic ketoacidosis (DKA).

3. Explain the patient's presenting signs and symptoms (S/S). (List six.)

CASE STUDY PROGRESS

Her current vital signs (VS) are 90/50, 124, 36 and deep, 101.3°F (tympanic).

4. Are these VS appropriate for a woman of C.J.'s age? Why or why not? Discuss your rationale.

5. A decision has been made to transport C.J. by ambulance to the local ED. After evaluating C.J., the ED physician writes the following orders. Carefully review each order. Mark with an "A" if the order is appropriate; mark with an "I" if inappropriate. For each order you mark as "I," explain why it is inappropriate and correct the order. In addition, identify any appropriate interventions that should be added to the list.

_____ 1. 1000 ml lactated Ringer's (LR) IV STAT

_____ 2. 36 units lente insulin and 20 units regular insulin SC now

_____ 3. CBC with differential; complete metabolic panel (CMP); blood cultures × 2 sites; clean-catch urine for urinalysis (UA) and culture and sensitivity (C&S); stool for ova and parasites, *Clostridium difficile* toxin, and C&S; serum lactate, ketone, and osmolality; arterial blood gases (ABGs) on room air

_____ 4. 1800-calorie, carbohydrate-controlled diet

_____ 5. Ambulate qid

_____ 6. Acetaminophen (Tylenol) 650 mg PO

_____ 7. Furosemide (Lasix) 60 mg IV push (IVP) now

_____ 8. Urinary output every hour

_____ 9. VS every shift

CASE STUDY PROGRESS
All orders have been corrected and initiated. C.J. has received fluid resuscitation and is on a sliding-scale insulin drip via infusion pump. Her latest glucose was 347 mg/dl.

6. What is the rationale behind using an infusion pump for the insulin drip?

7. C.J. is ready for transport to the medical ICU. C.J.'s mother is beginning to realize that C.J. is more acutely ill than she thought. She leaves the room and begins to cry. How would you handle this situation?

8. C.J.'s mother asks where she can get more information on how C.J. can control her diabetes. What are some resources she may find useful?

CASE STUDY PROGRESS
C.J. is transported to the MICU in slightly improved condition. She continues to improve and is discharged from the hospital 3 days later.

Case Study **145**

Scenario

T.R. is a 22-year-old college senior who lives in the dormitory. His friend finds him wandering aimlessly about the campus appearing pale and sweaty. He engages T.R. in conversation and walks him to the campus medical clinic, where you are on duty. It is 1050. The friend explains to you how he found T.R. and states that T.R. has diabetes mellitus (DM) and takes insulin. T.R. is not wearing a medical warning tag.

1. What do you think is going on with T.R.?

2. What is the first action you would take?

3. Because the glucometer reading is 50 mg/dl, what would your next action be?

4. When you enter the room to administer the juice, T.R. is unresponsive. What should your next action be?

5. T.R. is breathing at 16 breaths/min, has a pulse of 85 beats/min and regular, but remains unresponsive. What should your next action be if (1) your clinic is well equipped for emergencies or (2) your clinic has no emergency supplies? Because this is an outpatient setting, your resources may vary.

CASE STUDY PROGRESS

A few minutes after dextrose is administered, T.R. begins to awaken. He becomes alert and asks where he is and what happened to him. You orient him, then explain what has transpired.

6. What questions would you ask to find out what precipitated these events?

CASE STUDY PROGRESS

T.R. tells you he took 35 units lantus insulin and 12 units of regular insulin at 0745. He says he was late to class, so he just grabbed an apple on the way. He adds that he has had two similar low-blood sugar episodes in the past. He treated them with candy and then ate a meal. He says he is on a 2000-calorie, carbohydrate (CHO)–controlled diet.

7. Based on your knowledge of different types of insulin, when would you expect T.R. to experience an insulin reaction?

8. List at least four important points that you would stress in discussing your teaching plan with T.R.

Case Study 146

Name ______________________ **Class/Group** ____________ **Date** ____________

Group Members ____

INSTRUCTIONS All questions apply to this case study. Your responses should be brief and to the point. When asked to provide several answers, list them in order of priority or significance. Do not assume information that is not provided. Please print or write clearly. If your response is not legible, it will be marked as ? and you will need to rewrite it.

Scenario

S.K., a 51-year-old roofer, is 180 cm tall and weighs 80 kg. He was admitted to the hospital 3 days ago after falling 15 feet from a roof. He sustained bilateral fractured wrists and an open fracture of the left tibia and fibula. He was taken to surgery for open reduction and internal fixation (ORIF) of all his fractures. He is recovering on your orthopedic unit. You have instructions to begin getting him out of bed and into the chair today. When you enter the room to get S.K. into the chair, you notice that he is agitated and dyspneic. He says to you, "My chest hurts real bad. I can't breathe."

1. Identify five possible reasons for S.K.'s symptoms.

CASE STUDY PROGRESS

You auscultate S.K.'s breath sounds. You find that they are diminished in the left lower lobe (LLL). S.K. is diaphoretic and tachypneic and has circumoral cyanosis. His apical pulse is irregular and 110 beats/min.

2. List in order of priority three actions you should take next.

CASE STUDY PROGRESS

The physician orders the following: arterial blood gases (ABGs), chest x-ray (CXR), ECG, and ventilation/perfusion (V/Q) lung scan. The blood gas results come back as follows (these results reflect values at sea level): pH 7.47, $Paco_2$ 33.6 mm Hg, Pao_2 52 mm Hg, HCO_3 24.2 mmol/L, base excess (BE) –3, Sao_2 83%, and alveolar-arterial (A-a oxygen) gradient 32 mm Hg.

3. What is your interpretation of the blood gases? Be prepared to give the rationale for your interpretations.

4. Based on the ABGs and your assessment findings, what do you think is wrong with S.K.?

5. The physician writes the following orders for S.K. Carefully review each order. Mark with an "A" if the order is appropriate; mark with an "I" if the order is inappropriate. Correct all inappropriate orders, and provide rationales for your decisions.

____ 1. Transfer to MICU

____ 2. Heparin 20,000 units IV push (IVP) now, and 20,000 units in 1000 ml/D_5W to run at 1000 units/hr

____ 3. PT/INR and PTT q4h; call house officer with results

____ 4. 3 L oxygen by nasal cannula (O_2/NC)

____ 5. Patient-controlled analgesia (PCA) pump with morphine sulfate: loading dose 10 mg; dose 2 mg; lock-out time 15 minutes; maximum 4-hour dose 30 mg

____ 6. Streptokinase 250,000 IU IV over 30 minutes, then 100,000 IU/hr × 24 hours

____ 7. Prednisolone (Solu-Cortef) 1 g IV now

____ 8. Albuterol (Proventil) metered-dose inhaler (MDI), two puffs q6h

CASE STUDY PROGRESS

All orders have been corrected. S.K.'s V/Q scan indicates a pulmonary embolism (PE) in the LLL, and heparin therapy is initiated. Repeat ABGs show the following values (these results reflect values at sea level): pH 7.45, $Paco_2$ 35 mm Hg, Pao_2 82 mm Hg, HCO_3 24 mmol/L, BE −2.4, Sao_2 90%, A-a gradient 28 mm Hg.

6. What do these gases generally indicate?

7. The physician orders furosemide (Lasix) 20 mg IV now. Why do you think the physician ordered furosemide for S.K.?

CASE STUDY PROGRESS

S.K. is watched closely for the next several days for the onset of pulmonary edema. Heparin therapy, oxygen, pulse oximetry, daily CXRs and ABG analysis, and pain management are continued. When he is stable, S.K. is transferred back to your orthopedic unit.

8. The next day S.K. suddenly explodes and throws the physical therapist (PT) out of his room. He yells, "I'm sick and tired of having everyone tell me what to do." How are you going to deal with this situation?

Case Study **147**

Name _____ Class/Group _____ Date _____
Group Members _____
INSTRUCTIONS All questions apply to this case study. Your responses should be brief and to the point. When asked to provide several answers, list them in order of priority or significance. Do not assume information that is not provided. Please print or write clearly. If your response is not legible, it will be marked as ? and you will need to rewrite it.

Scenario

D.V. is a 38-year-old woman diagnosed with a ruptured appendix. She developed peritonitis and was discharged 9 days later with a left peripherally inserted central catheter (PICC) to home care for IV antibiotic therapy. You work for the home care department of the hospital. You have been assigned to D.V.'s case, and this is your first home visit. You are to do a full assessment on D.V. During the assessment, you notice a large ecchymotic area over the right upper arm. You ask her if she fell and hit her arm. She tells you, "The nurses took my blood pressure [BP] so many times it bruised."

1. Do you accept D.V.'s explanation? Why or why not?

2. In examining D.V. further, you find a fine, nonraised, dark red rash over her trunk (petechiae). What questions would you ask D.V. to elicit additional information?

CASE STUDY PROGRESS

D.V. hadn't noticed the petechiae before you pointed it out. The rash does not itch or cause pain. She has never had one like it before.

3. What other information would you want to gather?

CASE STUDY PROGRESS

The wound is not discolored or draining; the abdomen is tender to palpation. There is oozing of sero-sanguineous fluid around the PICC insertion site. The rash is confined to the trunk. You make a decision to call the physician regarding your findings.

4. What vital information will you relay to the physician? (Always start by identifying yourself.)

CASE STUDY PROGRESS

The physician orders blood to be drawn for coagulation studies and a CBC with differential. He says he would like to evaluate D.V. for disseminated intravascular coagulation (DIC).

5. What laboratory tests would you expect to see performed in coagulation studies?

CASE STUDY PROGRESS

You give D.V. her antibiotic, draw her blood, and take it to the lab. You return 6 hours later to administer another dose of antibiotics. D.V. greets you at the door. She is upset and ushers you to the bathroom, where you find blood in the toilet. She tells you that she has been urinating blood for the past 2 or 3 hours. She also shows you a tissue in which she has bloody-appearing sputum. She tells you she has been coughing up blood and shows you the bloody drainage from the blood draw 6 hours earlier. You notify the physician, who instructs you to call 911 and get the patient to the emergency department (ED) immediately. You call the ED and give report to the triage nurse on duty.

6.   What are you going to tell the triage nurse?

7.   Are the patient's presenting signs and symptoms (S/S) consistent with DIC? Explain.

CASE STUDY PROGRESS

The following labs were prolonged: PT/INR, PTT, split fibrin products, and D-dimer specifically. The following labs were decreased: platelets, platelet aggregation time, clot retraction time, and fibrinogen level. The WBC was 12.5 thou/cmm, and platelet count 46 thou/cmm. D.V. is diagnosed with DIC.

8.   List at least three priority needs for D.V.

CASE STUDY PROGRESS

D.V. is stabilized with oxygen, fluids, and blood products, and medication therapy is initiated. She is transferred to the ICU in guarded condition.

✻ **Note:** *The prognosis for someone with DIC depends on treating the underlying cause—in this case, her peritoneal infection.*

Case Study **148**

Name _____ Class/Group _____ Date _____
Group Members _____
INSTRUCTIONS All questions apply to this case study. Your responses should be brief and to the point. When asked
to provide several answers, list them in order of priority or significance. Do not assume information that is not provided.
Please print or write clearly. If your response is not legible, it will be marked as ? and you will need to rewrite it.

Scenario

You are the trauma nurse working in a busy tertiary care facility. You receive a call from the paramedics that they are en route to your facility with the victim of multiple gunshot wounds to the chest and abdomen. The paramedics have started two large-bore IV lines with lactated Ringer's (LR) and oxygen (O$_2$) by mask at 15 L/min. The patient has a sucking chest wound on the left and a wound in the right upper quadrant (RUQ) of the abdomen. Vital signs (VS) are 80/36, 140, 42. The patient is diaphoretic, very pale, and confused. Their estimated time of arrival (ETA) is 4 minutes.

1. List at least six things you will do to prepare for this patient's arrival.

CASE STUDY PROGRESS
On arrival to the emergency department (ED), your patient, B.W., is cyanotic and in severe respiratory distress. When he is transferred to the trauma stretcher, you notice that there is an occlusive dressing over the sucking chest wound. It is taped down on all sides.

2. Is taping the occlusive dressing on all sides appropriate? Explain.

3. Who usually responds to a trauma code, and what are the functions of the people from the various departments?

� **4.** Prioritize the actions of the physicians and nurses in the trauma situation.

5. B.W. is to have a CT scan of the abdomen. His abdomen has become distended and rigid. What are the possible reasons for the abdominal distention and rigidity?

CASE STUDY PROGRESS

The abdominal CT scan shows a large liver laceration. B.W. will be taken directly to the operating room (OR) for an exploratory laparotomy with repair of liver laceration, then to the ICU. When you return from transporting the patient to the OR, B.W.'s wife is in the ED, upset and frightened. The social worker has been called to another emergency.

6. How would you interact with B.W.'s wife?

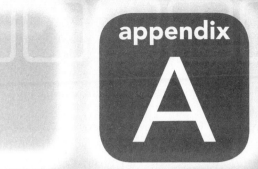

appendix A

Pointers for Students: How to Look Like You Know What You're Doing

Clinical experiences can be overwhelming and confusing; the environment is filled with distractions. What you experience often doesn't resemble what you have read in the book! We want to help you become a good clinician. The following are "tips and tricks" contributed by the writers of these cases. They are presented in no particular order of importance. Don't read all of them at once; read a few here and there, think about them, and apply them as you get the opportunity.

General Suggestions

- There are 5 instruments every nursing student should carry at all times. Never lend these items to anyone unless you can afford to replace them without complaint. These 5 essential items are a good black-ink ballpoint pen; a high-quality stethoscope; a pocket penlight (preferably with pupil sizes or centimeter ruler on the side); a medium-sized hemostat (straight Kelly); and a pair of bandage scissors.
- Purchase a high-quality stethoscope. Try listening with several different types, and choose the one that is best for you. Engrave your name on it. Your stethoscope is a very important tool.
- Staying hydrated will help you stay more alert. Drink plenty of fluids. (Besides the health benefits, this gives you an excuse to go to the bathroom for 30-second breaks!)
- Keep a quick snack handy. Sometimes you need a pick-me-up and don't have time for meals or to leave the unit to get something.
- Plan something special you can do to help alleviate stress—and use it on a regular basis.
- Avoid use of slang or words that could offend patients and families. Be aware of your patient's comfort level. Do not call patients by their first name unless they have given you permission.
- Assume nothing and take nothing for granted.
- Listen and observe carefully. Be aware of changes and try to assess their significance.
- Watch how the nurses you work with do things, and pick out things that work best for you.

- You can also learn from a negative example. If nothing else, you learn how *not* to do something!
- Projecting confidence and a "matter of fact" manner will usually put the patient, and yourself, at ease.
- Take care to respect each patient's confidentiality. Conduct interviews and examinations in a private and professional manner.
- Watch for physical or emotional scars. Health care touches on the most intimate experiences of our lives. Individuals—both men and women—who have been subjected to the degradation of sexual abuse and molestation may be especially prone to shame, aversion, or aggressive reactions.
- Don't be surprised when you discover that many adults are not knowledgeable about the basics of elimination and sexual functioning. Their ignorance or discomfort often is covered up with humor or aggressive behavior.
- It is imperative to give patients written instructions and information. It is critical that patients be able to understand the information and follow the instructions. Therefore, patient handouts should be developed using fonts that are a bit bigger than average and easy to read, and the text should be written at a sixth grade level of comprehension.
- If you have a limited budget and a clinical setting of patients who speak more than one language, ask for volunteers to help translate educational material—and then have that work double-checked. Local ethnic clubs or support groups can be a good source of translators.
- Never trust equipment. Don't assume anything. Equipment tends to break down at the worst times. Double-check to be certain all equipment is functional.
- Treat the patient, not the monitoring devices, numbers, or diagnosis.
- Not every patient with hepatitis or cirrhosis is an alcoholic.
- Not every alcoholic will go into delirium tremens.
- Do not assume patients are anorexic just because they look malnourished.
- Do not assume patients are well nourished just because they are obese.

Assessment and Data Collection

- Learn to assess pain without leaving out important data. Suggestion: use the COLDERRA method where C = characteristics, O = onset, L = location, D = duration, E = exacerbation, R = relief, R = radiation, and A = associated signs and symptoms.
- Begin with the basics and keep reviewing them: airway, breathing, circulation (ABCs).
- When you see acute changes in level of consciousness, first check oxygenation status.
- Become a keen observer; use all your senses.
- Be sensitive to hesitation and nonverbal cues when gathering information. What is left unsaid may be extremely important. Use phrases such as "Could you tell me more?" or "Could you help me understand?" to elicit more information.
- Don't be distracted by the obvious. Keep looking!
- Formulate a systematic way of assessing patients, and make it a habit. Go through the same sequence every time. You will be less likely to overlook or omit something.
- You can't find something if you don't look for it.
- Don't trust (1) machines, (2) numbers, or (3) what you can't see.
- Occasionally ask an experienced nurse or instructor to watch you do your assessments. Everyone, no matter how experienced, can benefit from objective suggestions for improvement. Over time, it is easy to become sloppy or start forgetting important things.
- With the first assessment of your shift, check the patient's ID bracelet and the rate and type of every fluid infusing—you are responsible for fluids under your control from the moment your shift begins until your shift is over.
- Remember to auscultate before palpating: Watch! Listen! *Then* Touch!

- Testing pH of nasogastric tube (NGT) drainage is easier if you slip the litmus paper into the end of the NGT and reconnect the tube to suction. Drainage will be pulled over the paper, which can then be removed. (Of course, antacids in the tube will negate this.)
- Any abrupt change in color or amount of drainage from wounds or drains needs to be explored and reported.
- Do not suggest words to describe feelings or events to your patients. You may miss subtle nuances if you jump to conclusions; listen to what your patients have to say and the words they use to say it.
- Perform a thorough psychosocial assessment that includes taking the values of patients and their significant others seriously.
- Include the significant others when you assess sleep patterns. They may be able to tell you more about snoring and other sleep disturbances than the patient can.
- Accurate recording of data, such as intake and output (I&O), is a must. Lawsuits have been won—and lost—over one single I&O sheet. Involve the patient and family in helping to keep accurate records. Ask them to let you know about foods or liquids brought in to the patient.
- Always double-check calculations; use a calculator, if necessary.
- Acute cardiovascular and musculoskeletal injuries require frequent evaluation and documentation of the 5 P's: pulse, pallor, pain, paresthesia, and paralysis. Deterioration of status in any of these variables may indicate a medical emergency and requires a rapid response.
- Be alert for substance abuse as an underlying diagnosis in individuals whose hospitalization is sudden and unanticipated. Many nurses have been injured by patients in undiagnosed withdrawal. This may be a particular risk in motor vehicle accidents (MVAs) or medical crises in which alcohol or drug use may be contributing factors.
- Often patients and families will deny the existence of mental illness or abuse because of stigma or ignorance. Ask about family violence (verbal or physical) or suicide very carefully.

Understanding the Problem or Diagnosis

- You have gathered your information; now look at it. Do you see any patterns? Do the data fit the history? Do all medications fit the diagnoses? Are all diagnoses accounted for in the medications?
- Ask the following questions:
     Do the data make sense in the context of this patient?
     Do the data create a complete picture?
     Do you need additional data?
- Use the data to formulate your list of patient problems.
- Prioritize specific problem statements, and guard yourself against distractions.
- Never think you are too smart to look something up.

Developing Strategies of Care

- Plan and coordinate care with your patient. By discussing interventions and priorities, you will learn more about your patient's value system.
- Educate the patient as you carry out this process; process and outcomes can and should be integrated. A better-educated patient is more prepared to cooperate with the medical and nursing care regimen.
- Always include relationships, cultural orientation, self-esteem, and emotional issues in planning care.
- Prevent infection. Teach your patients and their families to wash their hands properly. Take them to the sink in the room and demonstrate handwashing techniques that you were taught in Nursing 101. Show them how to use a paper towel to turn off the faucet. Have them practice.

- Watch other health care providers to ensure they wash their hands. If you are training others who are with you, leave the water running in the sink as you leave the room—it is a strong hint for them to wash their hands as they follow you out!
- Check equipment; double-check if you have any doubts. You are responsible for reporting equipment that is not in working order. Equipment not in working order can result in shock or other forms of injury to personnel, patients, or families. Remove it from the room promptly, label it clearly with a brief description of what is wrong, and report it according to policy.
- Substance abuse is not an uncommon complication in the recovery of trauma patients. Consider a psychiatric nurse practitioner or social services consultation if you suspect this is a problem.
- Accidents or injuries can aggravate feelings and memories associated with earlier experiences of trauma and abuse. If responses to current health problems seem to be unusual or in excess of what is expected, consider consulting a psychiatric nurse practitioner or someone from social services.

Carrying Out the Care Plan
- Frequently check your patient's charts for STAT orders.
- Document everything you do; if it isn't charted, you didn't do it.
- Document the patient's response to treatments, medications, and activities.
- Let the patient's values and preferences guide you.
- Get the family and significant others to help, if appropriate.
- As the patient's resting respiratory rate doubles from baseline, he or she will need to be intubated and placed on mechanical ventilation.

Evaluation and Reevaluation
- Monitor carefully for changes, whether dramatic and sudden, or subtle and gradual.
- Include the patient and families in helping to evaluate care. Ask, "Do you feel that what we are doing is helping you? What do you think?"
- Is the patient getting better? If so, continue with the plan. If not, reassess and revise the plan as needed.
- Evaluate patient and spousal cooperation. Never label patients as "noncompliant." Determine why patients do not take their medication, complete treatments, etc. Perhaps the side effects of treatment make patients feel worse than the disease, and they are exercising their right of choice. Remember, "noncompliance" on the part of patients is more often "knowledge deficit" or ignorance on our part! Noncompliance is rare when there is true teamwork, and it is a misleading term. *Adherence* is a better, less judgmental word.
- Long-term problems, particularly fatigue and pain, often contribute to depression.
- Involve other health care professionals and pain specialists in addressing complex issues.

Teamwork Is the Key to Survival
- When you graduate and start working as a nurse, you will be expected to be a team leader, coordinating the patient care given by certified nursing assistants, other nurses, and students, with the care given by many other professionals. Use this opportunity to observe the nurses you think are the most effective in promoting teamwork. Analyze why they are effective, and try integrating those techniques into your own practice.
- Work at developing good relationships with other professionals. The health care system is complex and constantly changing. We all need and deserve respect. We also depend on one another.

Pointers for Students: How to Look Like You Know What You're Doing

- Getting to know the medical nutritionists (dietitians), pharmacists, physical and occupational therapists, psychologists, social workers, case managers, laboratory personnel, nurse practitioners, medical staff, pastoral counselors, and other professionals in your setting can make things a lot easier for you later on. While you are a student, learn as much as you can about the role of each professional and the most effective ways to interact with them. It all adds up to good patient care.
- Patient care settings can be stressful, high-pressure environments, especially in emergency situations. Some of the most important things you can remember are:

  Try to sort out the difference between fact and feelings.

  Be forgiving.

  Never take anything personally.

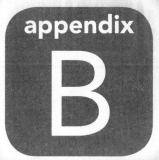

appendix B

Case Study Worksheet

Name _____ Chapter _____ Case _____ Date _____
Patient initials _____

Symbols/terms/abbreviations	Meaning/definition (diagnoses and medications go in following sections)
_____	_____
_____	_____
_____	_____
_____	_____
_____	_____
_____	_____
_____	_____
_____	_____

Diagnoses/medical conditions (+current and −past)	Description/meaning of diagnosis or medical problem (include possible significance)
_____	_____
	_____
_____	_____
	_____
_____	_____
	_____
_____	_____
	_____
	_____
	_____
	_____

Case Study Worksheet

Medications (brand and generic name if applicable)	Class, indications, contraindications, significant side effects, food and drug interactions
_____	_____
	_____
_____	_____
	_____
_____	_____
	_____
_____	_____

Treatments, interventions, and therapeutic procedures	Method of delivery, purpose/desired outcome, indications, contraindications, and precautions (include supplemental oxygen, tube feedings, therapeutic beds, etc.)
_____	_____
_____	_____
_____	_____
_____	_____

Laboratory tests and diagnostic procedures	What is it, when was it done, and why?
_____	_____
_____	_____
_____	_____
_____	_____
_____	_____
_____	_____
_____	_____

Cultural issues and their significance

_____	_____
_____	_____
_____	_____
_____	_____
_____	_____

Notes: _____

_____

_____

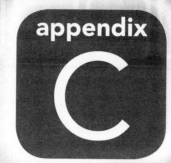

Abbreviations and Acronyms

AA	Alcoholics Anonymous	Alk Phos	alkaline phosphatase
AAA	abdominal aortic aneurysm	ALL	acute lymphoblastic leukemia
A-a gradient	alveolar-arterial oxygen gradient	ALP	alkaline phosphatase (serum)
		ALS	amyotrophic lateral sclerosis
AAO	awake, alert, and oriented	ALT (SGPT)	alanine transaminase (serum glutamic pyruvic transaminase)
ABCs	airway, breathing, circulation check(s)		
		AM	morning
ABGs	arterial blood gases	AMA	against medical advice
ABI	ankle-brachial index	AML	acute myelogenous leukemia
ac	before meals	ANA	antinuclear antibody
ACD	anemia of chronic disease	ANC (AGC)	absolute neutrophil count
ACEI	angiotensin-converting enzyme inhibitor	Anti-Sm	anti-smooth muscle antibody
		aPTT	activated partial thromboplastin time
ACh	acetylcholine		
AChR	acetylcholine receptor	ARB	angiotensin II receptor blocker
ACTH	adrenocorticotropic hormone	ARDS	adult respiratory distress syndrome
AD	autonomic dysreflexia		
ADA	American Dietetic Association; American Diabetes Association	AS	aortic stenosis
		ASA	aspirin
ADH	antidiuretic hormone	ASAP	as soon as possible
ADL	activities of daily living	AST (SGOT)	aspartate transaminase (serum glutamic oxaloacetic transaminase)
ad lib	as directed		
A-fib	atrial fibrillation		
AGC (ANC)	absolute granulocyte count	ATB	antibiotic
AGEs	advanced glycosylated end products	AV	atrioventricular; arteriovenous
		AVS	aortic valve stenosis
AIDS	acquired immunodeficiency syndrome	A&W	alive and well
		BAL	blood alcohol level
AKA	above-the-knee amputation	BE	base excess

bid	twice daily	CMP	complete metabolic panel (profile)
BiPAP	CPAP with mask over both mouth and nose	CMS	circulation, movement, sensation
BM	bowel movement	CMV	cytomegalovirus
BMI	body mass index	CNA	certified nursing assistant
BMP	basic metabolic panel	CNS	central nervous system
BNP	brain natriuretic peptide	CO	cardiac output; carbon monoxide
BOW	bag of waters		
BP	blood pressure	C/O	complaint(s) of, complaining of
BPH	benign prostatic hyperplasia		
bpm	beats per minute	CO_2	carbon dioxide
BR	bed rest	COPD	chronic obstructive pulmonary disease
brady	bradycardia		
BRB	bright red blood	CPAP	continuous positive airway pressure
BRP	bathroom privileges		
BS	bowel sounds; breath sounds	CPP	cerebral perfusion pressure
BSC	bedside commode	CPR	cardiopulmonary resuscitation
BSE	breast self-examination	CRF	chronic renal failure
BSF	basilar skull fracture	CRP	C-reactive protein
BUN	blood urea nitrogen	C&S	culture and sensitivity
Bx	biopsy	CSF	cerebrospinal fluid
CABG	coronary artery bypass graft	CT	chest tube
CAD	coronary artery disease	CTA	clear to auscultation
C&DB	cough and deep breathe	CT scan	computed tomography scan
cap	capsule	CV	cardiovascular
CAP	community-acquired pneumonia	CVA	cerebrovascular accident; costovertebral angle
CBC	complete blood count	CVC	central venous catheter
CBC with diff	complete blood count with differential	CVP	central venous pressure
		CWOCN	certified wound, ostomy, continence nurse
CBD	common bile duct		
CBG	capillary blood gas	CXR	chest x-ray
CBR	complete bed rest	DA	dopamine
C/C	chief complaint	DBP	diastolic blood pressure
CCU	coronary care unit	DC; D/C	discontinue
CDC	Centers for Disease Control and Prevention	DD	down drain
		DEXA scan	duel-energy x-ray absorptiometry
CDE	certified diabetes educator		
CEA	carcinoembryonic antigen	DI	diabetes insipidus
CHF	congestive heart failure	DIC	disseminated intravascular coagulation
CHO	carbohydrate(s)		
Chol	cholesterol	DKA	diabetic ketoacidosis
CI	cardiac index	DM	diabetes mellitus
CK (CPK)	creatinine phosphokinase	DME	durable medical equipment
CK-MM, CK-MB	CK isoenzymes	DNA	deoxyribonucleic acid
		DO	doctor of osteopathy
CLL	chronic lymphocytic leukemia	DOB	date of birth
CM	case manager	DOE	dyspnea on exertion
CML	chronic myelogenous leukemia		

Abbreviations and Acronyms

DPT	diphtheria, pertussis, tetanus	FHR	fetal heart rate
DSA	digital subtraction angiography	Fio$_2$	fraction of inspired oxygen
DSM-IV-TR	*Diagnostic and Statistical Manual of Mental Disorders*, 4th ed., text rev	FSH	follicle-stimulating hormone
		F/U	follow-up
		FUO	fever of unknown origin
D/T; d/t	due to	Fx	fracture
DTs	delirium tremens	GBS	Guillain-Barré syndrome
DTRs	deep tendon reflexes	GCS	Glasgow Coma Scale
DVT	deep vein thrombosis	GDM	gestational diabetes mellitus
Dx	diagnosis	GERD	gastroesophageal reflux disease
EBL	estimated blood loss	GFR	glomerular filtration rate
EC	emergency contraception	GGT	gamma-glutamyl transferase (transpeptidase)
ECF	extended care facility		
ECG	electrocardiogram	GH	growth hormone
echo	echocardiogram; cardiac ultrasound (sonogram)	GI	gastrointestinal
		GTT	glucose tolerance test
Ecoli	*Escherichia coli*	GU	genitourinary
ECT	electroconvulsive therapy	GXT	graded exercise (stress) test
ECU	emergency care unit	HA	headache
ED	emergency department; erectile dysfunction	HAV	hepatitis A virus
		Hb A$_{1c}$	hemoglobin A$_{1c}$; glycosylated hemoglobin test
EDC	estimated date of confinement		
EEG	electroencephalogram	HBAg	hepatitis B antigen
EF	ejection fraction	HBV	hepatitis B virus
EGD	esophagogastroduodenoscopy	hCG	human chorionic gonadotropin
EIA	enzyme immunoassay; exercise-induced asthma	HCl	hydrochloric acid
		HCO$_3$	bicarbonate ion
ELISA	enzyme-linked immunosorbent assay	Hct	hematocrit
		HCTZ	hydrochlorothiazide
EMG	electromyogram	HCV	hepatitis C virus
EMS	emergency medical system	HD	hemodialysis
EMT	emergency medical technician	HDL	high-density lipoprotein
EOMs	extraocular movements	HEENT	head, eyes, ears, nose, throat
EPS	evoked potential studies	HELLP	hemolysis, elevated liver enzymes, low platelets
ER	estrogen receptor		
ERCP	endoscopic retrograde cholangiopancreatogram	Hem/Onc	hematology/oncology
		HF	heart failure
ESP	erythropoietin-stimulating protein	Hgb	hemoglobin
		HgS	hemoglobin S
ESR	erythrocyte sedimentation rate	H/H	hemoglobin/hematocrit
ESRD	end-stage renal disease	HHH	hypervolemia, hypertension, hemodilution
ET	enterostomal therapist		
ETOH	alcohol	HIPAA	Health Insurance Portability and Accountability Act
ETT	endotracheal tube		
EVD	extraventricular drain	HIV	human immunodeficiency virus
FBG	fasting blood glucose		
FDA	U.S. Food and Drug Administration	HLA	human leukocyte antigen
		HMO	health maintenance organization
FFP	fresh frozen plasma	HO	house officer (physician)

HOB	head of bed	LBBB	left bundle branch block
HPV	human papillomavirus	LDH	lactate dehydrogenase
HRT	hormone replacement therapy (estrogen and progesterone)	LDL	low-density lipoprotein
		LE	lower extremities
HTN	hypertension	LES	lower esophageal sphincter
Hx	history	LFTs	liver function tests
IADLs	instrumental activities of daily living	LH	luteinizing hormone
		LLL	left lower lobe (of lungs)
IBD	inflammatory bowel disease	LLQ	left lower quadrant (of abdomen)
IBS	irritable bowel syndrome		
ICD; AICD	implantable cardioverter defibrillator; automatic ICD	LMP	last menstrual period
		LOC	level of consciousness
ICP	intracranial pressure	LPN	licensed practical nurse
ICS	intercostal space	LR	lactated Ringer's or Ringer's lactate
ICU	intensive care unit		
ID	identification	LUQ	left upper quadrant (of abdomen)
IDCA	idiopathic dilated cardiomyopathy		
		LV	left ventricle
IFG	impaired fasting glucose	LWS	low wall suction
IGT	impaired glucose tolerance	MAE(W)	moves all extremities (well)
IICP	increased intracranial pressure	MAOI	monoamine oxidase inhibitor
IM	intramuscular	MD	doctor of medicine
INR	International Normalized Ratio	MDI	multiple-dose injection; metered-dose inhaler
I&O	intake and output	meds	medications
IS	incentive spirometer	MG	myasthenia gravis
IT	intrathecal	MI	myocardial infarction
IUD	intrauterine device	MICU	medical intensive care unit
IV	intravenous	MNT	medical nutrition therapy
IVDA	intravenous drug abuse	MOM	milk of magnesia
IVF	intravenous fluid	MRI	magnetic resonance imaging
IVIg	intravenous immunoglobulin	MS	multiple sclerosis
IVP	intravenous push; intravenous pyelogram	MSOF	multiple system organ failure
		MUGA	multiple gated acquisition
IVPB	intravenous piggyback	MVA	motor vehicle accident
JNC	Joint National Committee on Prevention, Detection, Evaluation, and Treatment of High Blood Pressure	MVI	multivitamins
		MVP	mitral valve prolapse
		MVS	mitral valve stenosis
		NAD	no acute distress
JP	Jackson-Pratt	NC	nasal cannula
JVD	jugular venous distention	NCV	nerve conduction velocity
KS	Kaposi's sarcoma	NG	nasogastric
KUB	kidney, ureters, and bladder x-ray	NGT	nasogastric tube
		NH_3	ammonia
KVO	keep vein open	NICU	neonatal intensive care unit
L	left	NKA	no known allergies
lab(s)	laboratory; laboratory tests	NKDA	no known drug allergies
LAD	left anterior descending coronary artery	NOS	not otherwise specified
		NPH	neutral protamine hagedorn (a modified insulin)
lb	pound(s)		

NPO	nothing by mouth	PEFR	peak expiratory flow rate
NS	normal saline	PEG	percutaneous endoscopic gastrostomy tube
NSA	normal serum albumin		
NSAIDs	nonsteroidal antiinflammatory drugs	PEJ	percutaneous endoscopic jejunostomy tube
NTG	nitroglycerin	PEN	parenteral-enteral nutrition
N/V	nausea and vomiting	Pen VK	penicillin VK
O_2	oxygen	peri	perineal (related to perineum)
OB	obstetric	PERRL(A)	pupils equal, round, and reactive to light (accommodation)
OB/GYN	obstetrician/gynecologist		
OCD	obsessive-compulsive disorder		
OFC	occipital frontal circumference	PET	positron emission tomography
OGTT	oral glucose tolerance test	PFM	peak flow meter
OHCS; 17-OHCS	17-hydroxycorticosteroids	PFT	pulmonary function test
		pH	negative logarithm of the hydrogen ion concentration—acidity/basicity of the blood
OR	operating room		
ORIF	open reduction and internal fixation	PHD	public health department
OS	oculus sinister; left eye	PICC	peripherally inserted central catheter
OSA	obstructive sleep apnea		
OT; OTR	occupational therapist (therapy); registered occupational therapist	PID	pelvic inflammatory disease
		PIH	pregnancy-induced hypertension
OTC	over the counter	PKU	phenylketonuria
P	pulse	PM	afternoon or evening
PAB	prealbumin	PMH	past medical history
PACs	premature atrial contractions	PMI	point of maximal impulse
$Paco_2$	partial pressure of carbon dioxide in arterial blood	PN	parenteral nutrition
		PO	by mouth
PACU	postanesthesia care unit	POD	postoperative day
PAF	paroxysmal atrial fibrillation	postop	postoperatively
Pao_2	partial pressure of oxygen in arterial blood	PPD	purified protein derivative (test for TB); packs per day (cigarettes)
Pap	Papanicolaou smear		
PAP	pulmonary artery pressure	PPI	proton pump inhibitor
PBMV	percutaneous balloon mitral valvuloplasty	PPS	postpolio syndrome
		PR	progesterone receptor
PCA	patient-controlled analgesia	PRBCs	packed red blood cells
PCI	percutaneous coronary intervention	PRCs	packed red cells
		preop	preoperatively
PCN	penicillin	prn	as needed
PCP	primary care provider; *Pneumocystis carinii* pneumonia	PSA	prostate-specific antigen
		PSH	past surgical history
PCWP	pulmonary capillary wedge pressure	PT; RPT	physical therapist (therapy); registered physical therapist
PD	Parkinson's disease	PT	prothrombin time
PE	pulmonary embolus	PTCA	percutaneous transluminal coronary angioplasty
PEEP	positive end-expiratory pressure		
		PTH	parathyroid hormone
PEF	peak expiratory flow	PTSD	posttraumatic stress disorder

PTT; aPTT	partial thromboplastin time; activated partial thromboplastin time	SLE	systemic lupus erythematosus
		SLP	speech–language pathologist
PUD	peptic ulcer disease	SNS	sympathetic nervous system
PVCs	premature ventricular contractions	SOB	short (shortness) of breath
		S/P	status post
PVD	peripheral vascular disease	S/S	signs and symptoms
PVR	postvoiding residual	SSRI	selective serotonin reuptake inhibitor
q	every (e.g., q2h)		
R	right; respirations	S/T	secondary to
RA	room air; rheumatoid arthritis	STAT	immediately
RAI	radioactive iodine	STD	sexually transmitted disease
RBCs	red blood cells	SVR	systemic vascular resistance
RCA	right coronary artery	T&A	tonsillectomy and adenoidectomy
RD	registered dietitian	tachy	tachycardic
RDS	respiratory distress syndrome	TAH	total abdominal hysterectomy
rehab	rehabilitation	TB	tuberculosis
REM	rapid eye movement	T&C	type and crossmatch
RHD	rheumatic heart disease	TCA	tricyclic antidepressant
RLL	right lower lobe (of lung)	Td	tetanus/diphtheria (vaccine)
RLQ	right lower quadrant (of abdomen)	TED	thromboembolic deterrent
		TF	tube feeding
RML	right middle lobe (of lung)	TIA	transient ischemic attack
RN	registered nurse	TICU	thoracic intensive care unit
RNA	ribonucleic acid	tid	3 times per day
R/O	rule out	TKO	to keep open
ROM	range of motion	TM	tympanic membrane
RPR	rapid plasma reagin (test for syphilis)	TPA	tissue plasminogen activator
		TPN	total parenteral nutrition
RSV	respiratory syncytial virus	Trig	triglycerides
RT	respiratory therapist (therapy)	TSH	thyroid–stimulating hormone
R/T	related to	TUMT	transurethral microwave thermotherapy
RUQ	right upper quadrant (of abdomen)	TUNA	transurethral needle ablation
SAH	subarachnoid hemorrhage	TURP	transurethral resection of the prostate
Sao_2	arterial oxygen saturation		
SBO	small bowel obstruction	Tx	treatment
SBP	systolic blood pressure	UA	urinalysis
SC	subcutaneous	UDA	urinary drainage apparatus
SCC	sickle cell crisis	UEs	upper extremities
SCD	sickle cell disease; sequential compression device	UGI	upper gastrointestinal
		UGIB	upper gastrointestinal bleed
SCI	spinal cord injury	UOP	urinary output
SD	standard deviation	UPPP	uvulopalatopharyngoplasty
sed rate	erythrocyte sedimentation rate	URI	upper respiratory tract infection
SES	socioeconomic status		
SIADH	syndrome of inappropriate antidiuretic hormone	URR	urea reduction ratio
		US	ultrasound
SICU	surgical intensive care unit	UTI	urinary tract infection
SL	sublingual	UVJ	ureteral vesicle junction

Abbreviations and Acronyms

VA	Veterans Administration	V-tach	ventricular tachycardia
VDRL	Venereal Disease Research Laboratory (test for syphilis)	WAS	withdrawal assessment scale
		WBCs	white blood cells
V-fib	ventricular fibrillation	W/C	wheelchair
VLDL	very-low-density lipoprotein	WHR	waist/hip ratio
VP	ventriculoperitoneal	WNL	within normal limits
$\dot{V}/\dot{Q}$ scan	ventilation-perfusion scan (of lungs)	WNR	within normal range
		W/O	without
VS	vital signs	yo	year-old
V_T	tidal volume	yoa	years of age